HOSPICE

Prescription for Terminal Care

Kenneth P. Cohen, Ph.D, MPH

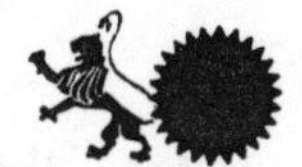

Aspen Systems Corporation
Germantown, Maryland
London, England
1979

Library of Congress Cataloging in Publication Data

Cohen, Kenneth P.
Hospice, prescription for terminal care.

Bibliography: p. 271.
Includes index.

1. Terminal care. 2. Terminal care facilities.
3. Terminal care facilities—United States. I. Title.
R726.8.C63 362.1 79-13341
ISBN 0-89443-151-X

Library of Congress Catalog Card Number: 79-13341
ISBN: 0-89443-151-X

Printed in the United States of America

1 2 3 4 5

Table of Contents

Foreword

Do not go gentle into that good night.
Rage, rage against the dying of the light.
Dylan Thomas

Rage and resistance are characteristic of the modern way of dying. Long before Dylan Thomas urged us to hold on to life tenacicusly, to our last breath, most people identified death as an intruder, a thief of existence, an unfair enemy to be bitterly fought.

Nowhere are these values more firmly and totally accepted than within the medical care system. Generations of health professionals have been taught that their duty is to preserve life with every skill and all the energy at their command. Time and time again, marvelous new discoveries appear on the scene to snatch people back from the jaws of death, further reinforcing this precept to save life at all costs. Unfortunately, the combination of this rapidly expanding technology, and health professionals' grim determination to use it to the fullest, frequently make patients' final death scenes unnecessarily difficult for all concerned—patients, families, and health professionals themselves.

In recent years, there has been a reaction against this tenacious clinging to life at all costs. A careful re-examination of the dying process, begun in England and now gradually moving to Canada and the United States, has led thoughtful health professionals in this country to explore interesting new approaches to death and the care of dying patients. Many, if not all, of these new approaches can be found in the various hospice programs now developing all over this country. Brought into existence by the new and burgeoning interest in the care of patients with terminal illnesses, these programs have in turn made contributions that have pushed back the boundaries of our knowledge and experience.

In this volume, Kenneth Cohen documents the phenomenal growth of hospice programs for the care of the dying in this country, and he points out many of the benefits and some of the hazards of that rapid growth. Moving from the early history of hospices in England, he traces the steady progression that has brought more than 250 hospices into existence in Great Britain, Canada, and the United States. He reports with considerable insight on the tremendous groundswell of interest in hospices and related programs among physicians, nurses, social workers, chaplains, hospital administrators, and others in the health care field.

We are, however, merely at the earliest beginning of a new era in the care of the dying, and many important questions remain to be answered. How many hospice programs does this country need to serve the dying? What kinds of programs are needed and where should they be based—in hospitals, in free-standing programs not related to hospitals, in home care programs, or in some combination of all three? How should these programs be financed? Where will the trained personnel be found—considerate and caring nurses, doctors, and others who are required to provide a *really* good program of hospice care? What new laws or legislation will be necessary to clarify and protect the interest of patients, their families, the health care providers who care for them, and society in general?

Dr. Cohen certainly does not provide all the final answers, since many of these questions are only now beginning to be asked, even by people who have worked in the field for some time. He does, however, begin an exploration of the issues, which will eventually lead to answers, and that is a very important beginning. I recommend *Hospice: Prescription for Terminal Care* to all people who are interested in the problems of death and dying, and I urge them to use it to build a better system of care for us all.

Paul R. Torrens, M.D., M.P.H.
Professor and Chairman
Division of Health Services
and Hospital Administration
School of Public Health
University of California, Los Angeles

Preface

The concept of hospice care for the terminally ill is a development of relatively modern times, although it has its origins in antiquity. Until now, the number of books on the subject could be counted on one hand. However, I predict that we are standing on the brink of a hospice information explosion. The hospice movement is in its infancy; as more hospices develop, their founders will publish accounts of their experiences for the guidance and information of new developers, who in turn will publish, and so the literature will expand at a geometric rate.

Because the hospice literature is still relatively sparse, I felt that an overview of the major issues was needed. This is not a how-to-do-it book. It is not a clinical treatise on death, dying, suicide, cancer, and pain control, although each of these issues is covered in varying depths. Rather, it is a journey through the maze of concepts, attitudes, philosophies, and rubrics surrounding the topic.

Some hospice advocates and others feel it inappropriate to mention euthanasia, the right to die, and suicide in a book about hospice. I feel that these are important issues surrounding the topic of death, dying, and hospice, and that they should be discussed to give the reader a complete picture of the overlapping issues. The reader is cautioned, however, not to equate euthanasia, the right to die, and suicide with hospice. Rather, hospice is a caring community, a program to care, compassionately, for terminally ill patients and their families.

This volume has been written for the general information of health care workers as well as legislators, insurance company executives, attorneys, clergy, educators, senior citizens, junior citizens, those interested in developing hospice programs in their communities, city planners, city managers—in short, anyone interested in the problems of caring for the terminally ill. Appendix A lists more than 250 hospices in the United States, Canada, and Great Britain. The listing includes both active hospices and those in various stages of development. Appendix B lists organizations to contact for more information regarding some of the issues covered. The glossary can be especially helpful to those not in the health care field.

Acknowledgments

As a hospital administrator, I have for years been surrounded, peripherally at least, by death. I have personally witnessed a number of in-hospital deaths of terminally ill patients. These scenes are not easily forgotten. Discussions with physicians, nurses, social workers, clergy and others regarding this kind of death gradually evolved into the basic concepts of this work. I have been influenced, consciously and perhaps unconsciously, by numerous individuals. I especially appreciate the ideas on death, dying, and the quality of life that were shared with me by Leonard Kovner, M.D., Chief of Surgery at Van Nuys Community Hospital, Van Nuys, California. More specific preliminary guidance on hospice development came through discussions with Paul Torrens, M.D., M.P.H., Professor and Chairman, Division of Health Services and Hospital Administration, School of Public Health, University of California, Los Angeles.

Many individuals too numerous to mention here aided in developing the philosophies and ideas in this volume. The knowledge gained from being a member of the Southern California Hospice Association, under the able chairmanship of Douglas McKell and later Dr. Edwin Olsen, was invaluable. All the members of that group helped, both directly and indirectly, to bring this project to fruition.

Finally, my family deserves kudos—especially Jeanette, who has been such a wonderfully supportive wife during all the years of study. She patiently withstood a seemingly endless number of evenings and weekends without my presence while I was engaged in research and writing.

Kenneth P. Cohen

Chapter 1

Hospice Versus Hospital Care

Death is the only thing we haven't succeeded in completely vulgarizing.
Aldous Huxley, *Eyeless in Gaza*

"Help me to die. Please give me something! I don't want to live like this. Please!" pleaded the frail Mrs. A., a mere wisp of a woman, confined to her hospital bed, fed intravenously, her respiration maintained by a mechanical respirator. The 82-year-old had been admitted two weeks earlier after x-rays showed a large carcinoma of the stomach. In spite of large doses of pain-killing drugs, including morphine PRN, she suffered constantly.

Just four days previously she had collapsed with a massive pulmonary embolism. The hospital's chief surgical resident had performed a successful pulmonary embolectomy. She recovered sufficiently to understand her physician's explanation of what had taken place. She requested that, if she had another cardiopulmonary collapse, no steps be taken to prolong her life, for the pain of the cancer was now more than she could endure. Members of her family concurred with this request.

But the hospital staff would not permit Mrs. A to die so easily. Her heart stopped again on three occasions during the night and each time was restarted artificially by the hospital's code-blue resuscitation team. Mrs. A's body lingered on for three weeks in a delicate balance between life and death. Her pleas to end it all were ignored by the hospital staff, who took all precautions to keep her alive despite her wishes to the contrary. Mrs. A was forcefully kept breathing, all her vital signs monitored. Finally, her heart stopped and, mercifully, could not be restarted despite all attempts of the code-blue team.

This story is hypothetical. Yet this same type of scenario is played out with live characters in many acute general hospitals every day. Patients like Mrs. A have to suffer the indignities of their terminal illnesses, often because their physicians have not been entirely honest with them.

Many physicians have found it extremely difficult to declare a patient terminally ill. This is understandable. The adage "where there is life there is hope" is an aphorism subscribed to by many people. To declare a patient terminally ill seems to be an admission that all hope is lost, and most health care personnel involved with the patient cannot face this possibility. Then too, most physicians have been trained to keep patients alive; to consider anything else would be an admission of failure. Thus, care of the terminally ill in U.S. hospitals has for many years not been differentiated from general acute care, which is the *sine qua non* of hospital care.

HOSPICE CARE FOR THE TERMINALLY ILL

In recent years, care of the terminally ill has begun to be recognized as a specialized medical modality. We are still faced, however, with the reluctance of many physicians to declare that their patients *are* terminal. At this point, the physician must admit that these patients will soon die, that further attempts to cure will be useless, and that the best treatment for both patients and families is to make the patients as comfortable as possible and to ease them into a peaceful death.

The concept of the hospice has come into its own only in recent years—in the past 5 years in the United States and in the past 30 years in Great Britain. Hospice involves the skilled and compassionate care of the dying and their families. The central issue is one of care versus cure, and since dying patients are not going to be cured, it seems logical that they be cared for compassionately. "It is an innovation in the sense that until only recently," wrote Robert Woodson, "the specialized palliative care of the dying patient was left largely to chance or the charge nurse."[1]

According to the *Hillhaven Hospice Medical Newsletter,* "the hospice philosophy is one of providing an environment in which to die, but not of actively prolonging life or accelerating death."[2] Douglas McKell, in a brochure describing a hospice workshop at UCLA, depicted hospice in this way:

> Hospice is a way of helping the dying and their loved ones to maintain the dignity and humanness of the dying process, receiving sophisticated medical and nursing care. For hospice the focus is on helping the dying live as fully as possible, rather than on the disease process. It is the dis-ease of dying that hospice care seeks to eliminate through the control of symptoms.[3]

Hospice is a *program* for the care of the terminally ill; it is not necessarily a facility. Hospice can be carried out as a home care program, as a separate free-standing facility, as a department of a general acute-care hospital, as a multidisciplinary team of care givers that serves the patients wherever they may be housed in a general acute-care hospital, or as a separate facility attached either physically or organizationally to a general hospital. Add to these separate models day-care services, outpatient services, and home care to arrive at a picture of the variable types of organizations that can be known as hospices.

This is not to imply that each of these models is mutually exclusive. Indeed, to be a true hospice, the organization must provide both inpatient and home care for its patients and patients' families. But many organizations develop from either a home-care or inpatient model and ultimately blossom into a true hospice providing full hospice services.

Throughout, any references made to a specific hospice *model* (e.g., inpatient model, home care model, etc.) should be construed to mean the organizational mode that the organization used to begin providing hospice services. The organization either subsequently expanded to include all hospice services or is in the process of doing so.

HOSPICE GOALS

Care of the dying represents a significant gap in our health care system. The void exists partly because acute-care hospitals are ill-suited to meet the physical and emotional needs of the dying, who must watch their own deterioration and the slow approach of death over a period of weeks or months. Such institutions are geared, instead, to cure patients and send them home as quickly as possible, to give efficient rather than individually optimized care.[4]

Hospices, on the other hand, treat the symptoms (physical, emotional, and mental) rather than the disease. For example, after assessing the physical pain a patient is suffering, a hospice team will consider the options of nondrug palliative therapies, non-narcotic analgesics, and, as a last resort, narcotic analgesics. Tranquilizers and antidepressants may also be prescribed to control psychological distress. Frequent changes of position, back rubs, and bathing are routine. X-rays, infusions, intubations, and temperature, pulse, and blood pressure readings—common medical management techniques in hospitals—are not routine.[5]

In a general hospital, the staff spends its time pursuing four basic goals: investigation, diagnosis, cure, and the prolongation of life.[6] Hospice goals differ markedly. In contrast to traditional medical goals, a major aim of a hospice program is palliation of symptoms so that patients can live out their lives as comfortably and meaningfully as possible.[7] Hospices seek to accomplish these four goals for dying people: relief from the distressing symptoms of their disease, the security of a caring environment, sustained expert care, and the assurance they and their families won't be abandoned.[8]

The National Cancer Institute, in a request for a proposal entitled "Implementation of the Hospice Concept," indicated that the goals of a hospice program are to—

- ease the physical discomfort of the terminal cancer patient by employing pharmaceutical and advanced clinical techniques for effective symptom control,
- ease the psychological discomfort of the terminal cancer patient through programs allowing for active participation in scheduled activities or periods of peaceful withdrawal as determined by the patient, and
- aid in maintaining the emotional equilibrium of the patient and the family as they go through the traumatic life experience of progressive disease and ultimately the final separation of death.[9]

With malignant disease, there are three admissible goals: to cure, to prolong life, and to palliate. Until now, considerable interest, concern, and financial resources have been directed towards curing patients and, if this is not possible, prolonging life. We must now seek ways to improve the treatment of those for whom improving the quality of life is the only appropriate goal.[10]

There is no doubt that some of the basic tenets of hospice are in subtle conflict with the everyday practice of modern medicine. Today's physicians routinely use complicated machinery and invasive techniques in diagnosing and treating the sick, and many feel that they must bring all the available technology into play at all times or be charged with neglect or even euthanasia.[11] However, there is nothing in the technological training of physicians that equips them to deal with questions of ethical, aesthetic, or human value.[12] Therefore, the question might be asked: should physicians alone make all the decisions regarding the care of the terminally ill patient, the course of treatment, and even the place where such treatment and care will be provided?

For most people entering the health care system, the classic goals of investigation, diagnosis, treatment, and cure are most appropriate, and the mainstream of medicine should, indeed, continue in this direction. However, we must remember that for some people this orientation is not appropriate, that a different care plan for the dying is required.[13]

Fatal illness is frequently complicated, requiring the services of many different medical specialists. Most treatments tend to be elaborate, extensive, and expensive; many families are economically destitute by the time death occurs.[14] Krant calls the process—requiring the services of many different medical specialists—"discontinuous special care-giving." Such treatment tends to push the family physician more and more into the background, and the patient loses the closeness of a stable, continuous medical figure.[15]

Hospital utilization review committees transfer many terminally ill patients from hospitals to nursing homes. Most nursing homes, however, are oriented toward custodial care of older people and are not staffed with sufficient professional medical staff to deal adequately with the difficult problems of severe pain. These institutions offer minimal opportunity for community experience between patients, staff, and families and often prefer to send their residents back to the hospital to die.[16]

Not everyone can or should die at home, but, currently, care for the terminally ill in most existing acute-care institutions and nursing homes ranges from inadequate to poor.[17] Many people prefer to die at home rather than in an institution, but our modern society has developed the posture that the terminally ill would be better served in a general hospital, where all resources are brought to bear on curative attempts to prolong life, rather than palliation, which is the emphasis of hospices.

THE SCOPE OF THE PROBLEM

In 1974, the gross national product of the United States exceeded $1.4 trillion, the highest in history. Health expenditures have been rising every year in absolute dollars and in 1974 reached almost 9 percent of the gross national product.[18] Medical care personal expenses accounted for nearly $75.8 billion of this amount.[19] Full-time and part-time medical and other health service employees exceeded 3.8 million.[20] These figures indicate the enormity of the health care industry in the United States.

The Aging U.S. Population

At the beginning of this century, death came to about 15 percent of all children in their first year, and to perhaps another 15 percent before adolescence. Nowadays, fewer than 2 percent die in their first year, and the great majority will live to be over 70. Life expectancy at birth has improved by perhaps two and a half times. Life expectancy at 70 has changed very little; it is now approximately 12 years.[21]

The mortality rate in the United States has declined since 1900. This has paralleled changes in the age composition of the population. The 1900 rate was 17.2 per 1,000. By 1954, it had dropped to 9.2, a record low, and in 1966, it stood at 9.5. The outstanding difference between the 1900 and

1966 rates lies in the greatly reduced number of deaths during the first year of life and, to a lesser extent, during the years after the age of 55.[22]

What these statistics mean is that the average age of the population is increasing. This has led to a changing emphasis in the health care of the population. With greater numbers of people in older age groups, health care providers are concentrating more on the illnesses of middle age and the infirmities of old age.

As J. Alsofrom, reporting in *American Medical News* has observed,

> by the end of this decade ten million people will be receiving treatment for cancer and, each year, 385,000 will die from that disease. Kidney disease will afflict eight million people in the next few years, and by the end of 1977, 54,000 will die from renal failure or its complications. Old age certainly will hit all of us. Now there are almost 23 million senior citizens (65 or older), and because of medicine's life-prolonging techniques and pills, this number can only grow larger. The longer people live, the greater potential exists that they will contract fatal lingering illnesses.[23]

Cancer

The great preponderance of patients cared for in hospice programs are cancer patients. This is so because of the nature of cancer with its mercurial characteristics, which in most cases has evaded cures.

> Of the 700,000 people in the United States who develop cancer each year, it is estimated that one in three is "cured," (i.e., free of disease five years after definitive treatment). Many "cured" cancer patients, as well as those who develop recurrent or metastatic disease require long-range rehabilitation and/or continuing care services.
>
> At the present "cure" rate, however, there remains a significant population of cancer patients who will not show marked improvement following major therapy, but, who will suffer recurrence, progression of disease, and who, after a period of continuing care, will die.[24]

In 1900, tuberculosis was the leading cause of death in the U.S.; heart disease ranked fourth and cancer ranked eighth. As treatment of infectious diseases improved, the number of deaths due to heart disease and cancer increased. Today, cancer is the second most frequent cause of death in the U.S.[25] Of every six deaths from all causes in the U.S., one is from cancer. In 1977, an estimated 382,000 Americans died of cancer. In

1976 it was 374,000. In 1975 it was 365,693. In 1974, 360,472 cancer deaths were reported by the U.S. National Center for Health Statistics.[26] In 1978 about 390,000 people will have died of the disease—1,070 people per day, about one every 80 seconds. Thus, the scourge relentlessly increases year after year.

Much of the financial burden of cancer is related to the need for hospital care. A 1974 study reported that a typical in-patient hospital stay for a cancer patient lasts an average of 16 days and costs (in terms of actual payments made to hospitals from all sources) about $1,400 per stay. Assuming there are 1.3 million cancer patients under hospital care each year in the U.S., $1.8 billion per annum would be expended solely for this service.[27] Every year the direct cost of cancer is over $3 billion, a cold figure that does not measure the victims' suffering and their families' grief.[28]

Larry Burke, Director of the National Cancer Institute's grant-funding arm, the Cancer Control and Rehabilitation Division, has estimated that the cost of cancer care today is $21,000 per patient for a two-year period. The most cost-effective way to die is in one's home. Figures show that 70 percent of the cancer patients in this country die in hospitals, 10 percent in nursing homes, and 20 percent in their own homes. It costs between $16 and $30 a day to die at home, and $154 a day, for room and board alone, to die in a hospital.[29]

Cancer patients must be regarded as people under a special and severe form of stress. Cancer is commonly perceived as an always-fatal and particularly loathsome disease, not "clean" and not uncomplicated like, for example, the frequently more fatal heart disease. In addition to the expectation of prolonged and intense pain, it carries the threat of disability and, even more frightening, of recurrence and death. Thus, cancer becomes an unusually stressful experience which disrupts the most important lifelong patterns of behavior.[30]

Orville Kelly, founder of Make Today Count (a mutual support group for people with life-threatening illnesses, their families and friends), has reported receiving over 25,000 letters and phone calls in two years. "Almost none of them complain about the physical suffering of cancer. It's the emotional problems they talk about—and financial worries, of course."[31] Similarly, hospice attempts to ease the emotional as well as the physical suffering of cancer.

Where Do People Die?

Assuming you could choose where you would die, barring accidental traumatic death, would you choose to die in an institution or in your home? Would you prefer to be hooked up to tubes, machines, and gadgets that would prolong your breathing (and possibly your agony), or would you ask to be tended in a familiar environment surrounded by family, friends, pets, and personal possessions?

People no longer die in their homes in the midst of their families. They now die in institutions, principally hospitals, extended care facilities, and nursing homes. At the turn of the century, in metropolitan areas, 75 to 80 percent of deaths took place at home.[32] Now, the reverse holds true, especially in the cities, where more than 75 percent of all recorded deaths take place in institutions.[33]

National statistics on deaths occurring in hospitals and institutions have been published several times. In 1937, when annual data were first available on the subject, 37 percent of all recorded deaths occurred in hospitals and institutions. In the years following 1937, there was a gradual but steady increase in the percentage until 1949, when 50 percent of all recorded deaths occurred in such places. After 1949, data are not available again except for 1958, when the percentage jumped to 61 percent. Thus, over a 21-year period, there was a sizable and steady increase in both the number and percentage of deaths occurring in hospitals and institutions.[34]

A study conducted by the United States Department of Health, Education, and Welfare revealed that of the 1.7 million people who died in the United States in 1961, about 72 percent had one or more episodes of hospital or institutional care in the last year of life.[35] Sixty-three of the average hospitalized decedent's last 365 days were spent in hospitals and institutions. This average was 45 days when all decedents, including those not hospitalized at the time of death, were considered.[36]

Proportionately more females than males received care in hospitals or institutions in their last year of life (76 percent as compared with 70 percent). This difference is accounted for primarily by women's more frequent use of resident institutions.

Twelve percent fewer nonwhite than white decedents were reported as having had hospital or institutional care. Care was less frequent for nonwhites in both short-stay hospitals and resident institutions.[37] Nonwhite people had a much lower episode rate per 1,000 decedents (942) than white people (1,232).[38]

Although only 28 percent of those who died in 1961 had no hospital or institutional care in the year before death, 39 percent were not in medical facilities at the time of death. Thus, 11 percent of all decedents were hospitalized at some time in the last year of life yet did not die in a hospital or an institution. Of deaths occurring in hospitals and institutions, 823,000 were in short-stay hospitals and 214,000 in resident institutions.[39]

About 665,000 people, or about 39 percent of all decedents, died outside of hospitals in 1961. Although they were not in hospitals or institutions at the time of death, 29 percent had some hospitalization experience in the last year of life. Seventy-three thousand of those 665,000 died of malignant neoplasms. Of this number, 74.8 percent had hospital or institutional care during the last year. Thus, those dying of malignant neoplasms experienced two and a half times more hospital or institutional experience during the last year of life, although at the time of death they might not have been in a hospital or institution.[40] Of those hospitalized who died of malignant neoplasms, 40 percent had only one episode of care.[41]

Of the estimated 1,229,000 decedents who had hospitalization experience during the last year of life, 62 percent had one episode of care, 22 percent experienced two episodes, and the remaining 16 percent had three or more episodes of care in a hospital or institution.[42]

When classified according to the ten leading causes of death in 1961, the decedents most likely to have been hospitalized in the last year of life were infants who died of certain diseases of infancy and of congenital malformations, and elderly people who died of malignant neoplasms. More than 90 percent of the decedents in each of these three cause groups had hospitalization experience.[43]

As Benjamin Franklin wrote, "in this world nothing is certain but death and taxes." But while death is a certainty that is seldom easy, it need not be the painful experience that it so often is. Death in a hospital or institution may be traumatic not only for the patient but for the family and friends as well. Death in a hospice program, either at home or in a hospice facility, can be a peaceful, even a welcomed way to end one's days.

NOTES

1. Robert Woodson, "The Concept of Hospice Care in Terminal Disease," in *Breast Cancer*, ed. J. M. Vaeth (Basel, Switzerland: Karger, 1976), pp. 161–79.
2. *Hillhaven Hospice Medical Newsletter*, Hillhaven Hospice, Tucson, Arizona, 1, no. 1(n.d.):2.
3. Douglas C. McKell, "Hospice Care—A New Concept for the Care of the Terminally Ill and Their Families," Workshop at UCLA Extension, Los Angeles, April 8–9, 1978.
4. J. Kohn, "Hospice Movement Provides Humane Alternatives for Terminally Ill Patients," *Modern Healthcare* 6 (September 1976): 26 ff.
5. Janet Plant, "Finding a Home for Hospice Care in the United States," *Hospitals* 51 (July 1, 1977): 53–62.
6. "The Hospice Movement," Unpublished Management Services Special Report (Newport Beach, California: Advanced Health Systems, Inc., October 1977).
7. Kohn, loc. cit.
8. Joan Craven and Florence S. Wald, "Hospice Care for Dying Patients," *American Journal of Nursing* 75 (October 1975): 1,816–22.

9. Attachment to personal letter to author from Lawrence D. Burke, Program Director for Rehabilitation Treatment, Rehabilitation and Continuing Care Branch, DCCR, HEW, National Cancer Institute, Bethesda, Maryland, December 15, 1977.

10. Balfour M. Mount, "The Problem of Caring for the Dying in a General Hospital; the Palliative Care Unit as a Possible Solution," *Canadian Medical Association Journal* 115 (July 17, 1976): 119–21.

11. Alice Kantor, "Focus on Hospice: Improving the Quality of Life that Remains," *St. Luke's Hospital Center News* (New York), n.d., pp. 3–4.

12. Robert S. Morison, "Dying," *Life and Death and Medicine: A Scientific American Book* (San Francisco: W. H. Freeman & Co., 1973), p. 40.

13. Sylvia Lack, "I Want To Die While I'm Still Alive," *Death Education* 1, no. 2 (Summer 1977): 165–76.

14. Melvin J. Krant, *Dying and Dignity: The Meaning and Control of a Personal Death* (Springfield, Illinois: Thomas, 1974), pp. 52–53.

15. Ibid.

16. D. G. McCarthy, "Should Catholic Hospitals Sponsor Hospices?" *Hospital Progress* 57 (December 1976): 61–5.

17. Kohn, loc. cit.

18. U.S. Department of Commerce, Bureau of Economic Analysis, *The National Income and Product Accounts of the United States, 1929–74, Statistical Tables* (Washington, D.C.: U.S. Government Printing Office, 1977), table 1.1, pp. 2–3.

19. Ibid., table 2.6, pp. 88–90.

20. Ibid., table 6.7, pp. 204–5.

21. Morison, p. 39.

22. Ibid., p. 42.

23. J. Alsofrom, "Hospice Way of Dying—At Home with Friends and Family," *American Medical News* 20 (February 21, 1977): 7–9.

24. Letter from Lawrence D. Burke, Program Director for Rehabilitation Treatment, Rehabilitation and Continuing Care Branch (DCCR), National Cancer Institute, HEW, December 15, 1977, RFP, p. 1.

25. David Levin et al., *Cancer Rates and Risks,* 2nd ed., HEW Publication No. (NIH) 75-691 (Washington, D.C.: U.S. Government Printing Office, 1974), p. 2.

26. American Cancer Society, *1978 Cancer Facts and Figures* (New York: American Cancer Society, 1977), p. 4.

27. Levin et al., p. 3.

28. Michael B. Shimkin, *Science and Cancer,* HEW Publication No. (NIH) 74-568, 2nd rev. (Washington, D.C.: U.S. Government Printing Office, 1973), p. 3.

29. Alsofrom, citing Burke.

30. Morton Bard, "The Psychological Impact of Cancer and Cancer Surgery," *Proceedings of the American Cancer Society's National Conference on Human Values and Cancer,* June 22–24, 1972 (Atlanta: American Cancer Society, 1972), p. 24.

31. Donald R. Pellman, "Learning to Live with Dying," *New York Times Magazine,* December 5, 1976.

32. Krant, pp. 9–10.

33. U.S. Public Health Service, *Vital Statistics of the U.S., 1958,* vol. II (Washington, D.C.: U.S. Government Printing Office, 1960).

34. U.S. Department of Health, Education, Welfare, Public Health Services, National Center for Health Statistics, *Hospitalization in the Last Year of Life—1961*, series 22, no. 1 (Washington, D.C.: U.S. Government Printing Office, September 1965), p. 3.

35. Ibid., p. 2.

36. Ibid., p. 2.

37. Ibid.

38. U.S. Department of Health, Education & Welfare, National Center for Health Statistics, *Episodes and Duration of Hospitalization in the Last Year of Life, U.S., 1961*, Series 22, No. 2 (Washington, D.C.: U.S. Government Printing Office, June 1966), p. 1.

39. HEW, *Hospitalization in Last Year of Life—1961*, p. 2.

40. Ibid., p. 5 et passim.

41. HEW, *Episodes and Duration, 1961*, p. 2.

42. Ibid., p. 4.

43. HEW, *Hospitalization in the Last Year of Life—1961*, p. 2.

Chapter 2

The Origins of Hospice

Whatever hath no beginning may be confident of no end.
Sir Thomas Browne, *Urn-Burial*

The word *hospital* is derived from the Latin *hospitalis,* meaning "of a guest" and *hospes,* meaning "a guest." The French *hospice* is derived from the Latin *hospitium,* which was a place in which a guest was received. The English word *hospital* comes from the Old French *hospitale,* as do the words *hostel* and *hotel,* all originally derived from the Latin. The etymology of *hospital, hostel, hotel,* and *hospice* shows that although these words are now used with different meanings, they were at one time used in the same sense.

THE EARLIEST HOSPITALS

Since the beginnings of civilization, people have offered their favorite remedies to relieve the sufferings of their ill neighbors. As civilization progressed from the individual family unit to collective family groups and then to the organized community, the community's responsibility for the welfare of the unfortunate within its ranks came to be recognized.

> The history of medicine and surgery dates from earliest ages, but hospitals as social institutions to which the sick of a community can be brought for treatment have a later origin. The story of the birth and evolution of the hospital portrays the triumph of civilization over barbarism and of altruism over egoism, the slow but certain upward struggle against individualism, and the progress toward an ideal characterized by interest in the welfare of the entire community.[1]

Much of the information contained in this chapter was derived from Malcolm T. MacEachern, *Hospital Organization and Management* (Berwyn, Illinois: Physician's Record Company, 1962). Referenced citations reprinted by permission of the publisher.

India and Egypt

Two ancient civilizations, India and Egypt, had crude facilities which today we might call hospitals. According to Indian literature in the sixth century B.C., Buddha appointed a physician for every ten villages and built hospitals for the crippled and the poor; his son built shelters for the diseased and for pregnant women. Hospitals existed in Ceylon as early as 437 B.C.[2]

> The most outstanding of the early hospitals in India were 18 institutions built by King Asoka (273–232 B.C.). These are historically significant because of characteristics similar to those of the modern hospital [or hospice]. The attendants were ordered to give gentle care to the sick, to furnish them with fresh fruits and vegetables, to prepare medicines, to give massages, and to keep their own persons clean. Hindu physicians . . . were required to take daily baths, keep their hair and nails short, wear white clothes, and promise that they would respect the confidence of their patients.[3]

In early Egypt medical treatment was usually given in the home, while therapy away from home was available in the temples, which functioned as hospitals by being also centers of faith healing. Faith healing at that time was not of the same status as Egyptian medicine, since they had developed a set of surgical and medical procedures. The Egyptian physician was also often a priest; science and magic were integrated and both were used in the treatment of patients.

We have labeled these early facilities hospitals, since curative efforts were often attempted there. Yet because the medical technology of that day was so primitive, they frequently functioned as today's hospices do. Often, the only treatment that could be offered patients was compassionate and tender caring—in essence, nursing care and TLC.

Greece and Rome

Early Greek and Roman temples were also used as hospitals, providing refuge for the sick.

> One of these sanctuaries, dedicated to Aesculapius, Greek god of medicine, is said to have existed as early as 1134 B.C. at Titanus. Ruins still attest to the existence of another, more famous Greek temple built several centuries later in the Hieron, or

> sacred grove, at Epidaurus. Here the sick were ministered to in body and soul. The medicaments prescribed were salt, honey, and water from the sacred spring. To speed the cure they had hot and cold baths. Gymnasia accommodating thousands of persons were used for gymnasiotherapy. Equally large outdoor amphitheaters provided amusement. Important in treatment were long hours of sunshine and sea air combined with pleasant vistas. There were libraries and rooms for visitors, attendants, priests, and physicians. What might be described as the first clinical records were the columns of this temple at Epidaurus, upon which were inscribed the names of patients, brief histories of their cases, and comments as to whether or not they were cured.[4]

These Aesculapia spread throughout Greece as well as the Roman empire. Some were simply spas, administering water cures, while others administered the therapy outlined by the leading physicians of the day. The modern outpatient clinic seems to have originated in that day, in *tabernae medicae,* where only the ambulant sick were treated.

The Early Christian Influence

Even though the evolution of science was a prime factor in the founding of hospitals, the first hospitals were actually an outgrowth of religion rather than of medicine. The doctrines preached by Jesus, emphasizing love and pity, gave impetus to the establishment of hospitals, which, with the advance of Christianity, became integral parts of the church. These Christian hospitals replaced those of Greece and Rome. Devoted entirely to care of the sick, they accommodated patients in buildings outside the church proper.

> The decree of Constantinople in 335 closed the Aesculapia and stimulated the building of Christian hospitals, which, during the fourth and fifth centuries, reached the peak of their development. Many were erected by the rulers of the period or by wealthy Romans converted to Christianity. Justinian was instrumental in building the great hospital of St. Basil at Caesarea in 369, a veritable community for the sick, the aged, and orphans. The following year saw the building of a Christian hospital at Constantinople, where two wealthy deaconesses nursed the sick. A prominent Roman matron, Tabiola, endowed a public hospital in Rome in 390. At Edessa, Hippo, and Ephesus still

> others . . . were founded by the Christians. By the year 500 most large towns in the Roman empire had erected such edifices. Nursing, inspired by religion, was gentle and considerate, but the medical precepts of Hippocrates . . . and the other early Greek physicians were unfortunately being discarded because of their pagan origin, while mysticism and theurgy became more prominent.[5]

For several centuries up to the Middle Ages, very few records of hospitals have been found. There were probably very few outside the Italian cities. In European towns, occasional almshouses sheltered some of the sick; inns along the Roman roads housed others. Apparently, no provision was made for the care of thousands of helpless paupers, former slaves who had been set free when Christianity was introduced into the Roman empire.

The Mohammedans

The Mohammedans were almost as diligent as the Christians in caring for the sick. In Baghdad, Cairo, Damascus, Cordova, and many other cities under their control, they provided ample, and frequently luxurious, hospital accommodations. Because he was interested in the health of his people, Harun al-Rashid, the calif of Baghdad (786–809), built an extensive hospital system, paying the physicians himself and not charging patients for the care rendered. In 1160, a traveler reported that he had found as many as 60 dispensaries and infirmaries in Baghdad alone. Mohammedan medicine flourished up to about the fifteenth century, and it is noteworthy that Mohammedan countries had asylums for the insane a thousand years before such institutions appeared in Europe.

> The people of Islam made a brilliant start in medicine, but the great promise which glowed in their early work in medical arts and in hospitalization was never fulfilled. Wars, politics, superstition, and a nonprogressive philosophy stunted the growth of a system which, nevertheless, had some influence upon hospital development.[6]

THE MIDDLE AGES

Religion continued to be the dominant influence in the establishment of hospitals during the Middle Ages. These institutions were, however, primarily ecclesiastical rather than medical. Physical ailments were treated to afford relief, but there was little attempt to cure. The soul, not the body, was the major concern. Through love and faith, the priests, attendants, and physicians sought to elevate and discipline character according to the teachings of Christianity.

During the Crusades, *hospitia*, or travelers' rests and infirmaries, began to spring up adjacent to monasteries to provide food and temporary shelter for weary travelers and pilgrims. Probably the most famous of these are the hospices of Great St. Bernard and Little St. Bernard, two high passes across the Swiss Alps. The Great St. Bernard Hospice, at an elevation of 8,110 feet, was founded in the 1000s by St. Bernard of Menthon. Here Augustine monks still offer refuge for travelers, and during the severe winter months, the monks and their famous St. Bernard dogs save the lives of many snowbound wayfarers as they have for nearly a thousand years. Many summer travelers continue to visit this hospice, which has room for over 300 guests. Little St. Bernard lies about 25 miles southwest of Great St. Bernard. Its hospice dates from 962 and is nestled in the pass at an elevation of 7,170 feet.[7]

During the Crusades, families would also welcome travelers and pilgrims into their homes because they brought news and stories of the outside world. Sometimes travelers would give their hosts gifts, but generally a host would be glad to share food and shelter with travelers just for the pleasure of their company. Homeowners were expected to house pilgrims according to their rank or station in life. Sometimes, people complained that the pilgrims were less interested in the religious aspect of their journeys than in the prospect of staying free in their hosts' homes.[8]

The Order of St. John of Jerusalem

The hospital movement grew rapidly during the Crusades, which began in 1096. MacEachern wrote that "pestilence and disease were more potent in defeating the crusaders than were the swords of the Saracens."[9] Therefore, a number of military hospital orders sprang up, and hospitals and hospices for the care of sick and exhausted crusaders were provided along all traveled roads and important river crossings. Probably the most famous of these military hospital orders was the Knights Hospitallers of the Order of St. John of Jerusalem.

> The purpose of the order from its inception (about 1065) was the care of the needy sick. At first there was no thought of its becoming military in character. However, one of the duties in the care of the sick is their protection from enemies, and the Knights early found it necessary to defend their hospitals against the

> enemies of their Faith. They were the first organized military medical officers, and they . . . bore their full share of danger on the field of battle.[10]

In a February 15, 1113 document that is, in effect, the foundation charter of the Knights Hospitallers, mention was made of seven "possessions," or facilities, in Syria and Europe: St. Gilles, Asti, Pisa, Bari, Otranto, Faranto, and Messina. These were apparently resthouses for pilgrims on their way to the Holy Land, with facilities for caring for any who might fall sick or be wounded. This document is perhaps the earliest reference to beds being provided for patients, and it even goes so far as to specify the length and breadth required. There was none of the crowding of two or more patients into one bed, as was so common in hospitals throughout the world as late as the eighteenth century.[11]

In 1311, the Knights built a hospital at Rhodes, but this structure was evidently provisional and insufficient, for in 1314 a decision was made to found and endow a hospital that would serve all people of all lands. Even this building was not large enough, and in 1478 a larger structure was completed. By 1510, the hospital was again so crowded that incurables could no longer be admitted and a place was provided for them outside.[12] As in other hospitals of the Middle Ages, the ones at Rhodes were not only for the care of patients, but also for the accommodation of pilgrims.[13]

The great hospitals of the Order of St. John at Rhodes and later at Malta were not the only institutions for the care of the sick maintained by the Knights. Commanderies were scattered from one end of Europe to the other, and nearly every one of them had facilities for the care of the sick. Also, the nuns of the Order of St. John of Jerusalem ran a hospice for women, known as the Hospice of St. Mary Magdalene.[14]

The order's first duty was support of pilgrims and care of the poor. Patients were not mere cases, as patients sometimes fear they are in certain modern hospitals, but beings entitled to love and respect. "Perhaps with our progress in the art and science of medicine," Hume reflects, "we have lost much of this old feeling, even though our methods of treating disease be so much more advanced."[15]

All hospitals of the Middle Ages were costly, often decorated with colorful tapestries and stained glass windows, but the interiors consisted for the most part of large, drafty halls with beds lining each side. A master or warden was usually in charge, assisted by lay brothers and sisters. A few of the better institutions were arranged on the ward plan, usually built in the shape of a cross. Floors were made of red brick or stone. Heat was provided by open charcoal braziers. The stained glass windows were decorative but let in little or no light or air. The only ventilation came from the cupola in the ceiling.[16]

The great Al-Mansur Hospital, built in Cairo in 1276, provides a striking contrast to the European institutions of the period.

> Equipped with separate wards for the more serious diseases, with out-patient clinics, and with diet kitchens, it had conveniences that a modern hospital might well envy. It provided music and storytelling for the sleepless, operated homes for the convalescent, and inaugurated a policy of giving each patient a small sum of money on his departure.[17]

Lazar Houses

Leprosy spread during the twelfth and thirteenth centuries, and the leper became a difficult problem. Dawson tells us that the leper was "driven from his fellows, he was the 'pariah dog', unwelcome and unadmitted to any dwelling, village or town."[18]

> At the boundaries of many parishes was placed a stone trough, known as the "leper stone," in which food was placed by the charitably minded inhabitants for the use of itinerant lepers. Itinerant they need must be: belled like goats; driven from village to village; living on doles of food; unsheltered, scorned, and expelled, many died of privation and cold, whilst others less fortunate, dragged out an existence made terrible both by disease and their social outlawry.[19]

In response to their pitiable condition, lazar houses (from Lazarus, the leprous beggar mentioned in Luke 16:20) began to spring up in profusion and supplied additional hospital facilities. These were crude structures, usually built on the outskirts of towns and maintained for segregation of the ostracized lepers rather than for their treatment. The patients were nursed by special attendants, members of the Order of St. Lazar. In England and Scotland there were at one time some 220 of these lazar houses, and in France and Germany about 2,000 existed in each of the two countries. They actually represented a great social and hygienic movement since they served to check the spread of epidemics by isolating the sufferers. To them may be credited the virtual stamping out of leprosy.[20]

Monks and Medicine

According to MacEachern, medical progress was stifled by a Church edict of 1163 forbidding the clergy to perform operations that necessitated the shedding of blood.[21] Since monks and clerics were in those times essentially the only ones who had any semblance of an education, they were usually the physicians. However, many aspects of medical practice—medical fees, for example—were inconsistent with the ideals of the clergy, and decrees were issued from time to time limiting their medical activities. Besides stopping the monks from practicing medicine, these decrees had the effect of lowering the status of the entire medical profession. As a consequence, surgery was taken over by the barbers, whose practice of applying the leech was their primary medical therapy. Thus, a shadow fell upon the profession of surgery.[22]

HOSPITALS IN THE NEW WORLD

The first hospitals in the New World were built by the Spanish in Mexico City (1524) and by the French in Canada (1639). Before the American Revolution, most colonial cities had their pest houses and almshouses to care for the communicably ill, the aged, and the indigent. There was a general tendency to lump together the physically handicapped, the sick, the socially unwanted, and the pauper.

Philadelphia was the site of the first incorporated hospital in America. Founded in 1751, Benjamin Franklin helped to design the structure, and in 1755 the hospital, quite modern in plan with a central administration unit and two wings, was opened to the public. Its first medical staff, consisting of three physicians, gave their services without remuneration for three years. Benjamin Franklin was its first clerk and served as president for the first two years.

As late as 1769, New York City, with nearly 300,000 inhabitants, was without hospitals. In 1771, a group of citizens formed the Society of the New York Hospital and obtained a grant to build. On a site of five acres, they built a model structure that had a maximum of eight beds to the ward, good ventilation, and all the known facilities for care of the sick. The hospital was captured by the British during the Revolution and was used by them as a barracks and military hospital.

With postwar reconstruction, the New York Hospital broadened its services. It began giving instruction in nursing, and in 1779 it also introduced vaccination to America and established an ambulance service.

During the period of the late 1700s and the early 1800s, a substantial number of today's prestigious medical centers were founded. Among these were New York City's Bellevue Hospital and Boston's Massachusetts General Hospital. The hospital movement continued to spread until every important town in the United States had a hospital.

The word *hospice,* as it was used in the past, did not precisely denote a *hospital,* as we now use the term. Among the earliest hospitals, it is difficult to draw a distinction between a true hospital and a place where the weary traveler might find rest and safety. Yet, throughout its 2,000-year development, while the nature of the hospice/hospital has evolved, its primary goal—to provide compassionate care—has remained unchanged.

NOTES

1. Malcolm T. MacEachern, *Hospital Organization and Management,* rev. 3rd ed. (Berwyn, Illinois: Physicians' Record Co., 1962), p. 1.
2. Ibid., p. 2.
3. Ibid.
4. Ibid., p. 3.
5. Ibid., p. 4.
6. Ibid., p. 5.
7. Franklin Erickson, "St. Bernard, Great, and St. Bernard, Little," *World Book Encyclopedia,* 1967.
8. H. B. Meek, "Hotel," *World Book Encyclopedia,* 1967.
9. MacEachern, p. 6.
10. Edgar E. Hume, *Medical Work of the Knights Hospitallers of Saint John of Jerusalem* (Baltimore: Johns Hopkins University Press, 1940), p. 3.
11. Ibid., p. 13.
12. Ibid., pp. 47–8.
13. Ibid., p. 51.
14. Ibid., p. 64.
15. Ibid., p. 58.
16. MacEachern, p. 7.
17. Ibid., p. 10.
18. Bernard Dawson, *The History of Medicine* (London: Lewis, 1931), p. 98.
19. Ibid., pp. 98–9.
20. MacEachern, p. 7.
21. Ibid., p. 9.
22. Ibid.

Chapter 3

The Case of the Terminally Ill Patient

The stroke of death is as a lover's pinch, which hurts, and is desir'd.
Shakespeare, *Antony & Cleopatra*

The physician who attends the terminally ill patient will abandon cure, a legitimate medical decision, but will never abandon care.[1] The compassionate physician will recognize that the patient deserves as much attention as the acute-care patient, but another dimension has crept into the picture; the family, the bereaved, the survivors, must now be considered part of the unit of care.

For the patient who has learned of a terminal condition, the first step in separation is the realization that the course of life is changing. First, there is the illness, then the fact that intensive treatment no longer is effective, then that the disease is spreading, and finally, that life appears to be a matter of months, not years, not decades.[2]

Robert Christensen, a registered nurse, who for several weeks was attending a terminally ill leukemia patient with a prognosis of just a few hours or days of life, was faced with a decision. The patient began hemorrhaging from mouth and nose, began to choke on the flow of blood, and stopped breathing. Without hesitation, Christensen applied mouth to mouth resuscitation and prevented the patient from immediately dying. The patient survived for three more days, and the family greatly appreciated Mr. Christensen's magnanimous act, which might have been considered beyond the call of duty. Christensen asked, "does caring for a patient stop when nothing more can be done medically, or does real caring really begin when there is nothing left but caring, love, and compassion?"[3]

IN HOSPITAL

Consider the case of Mrs. B., in her late seventies, who had suffered a stroke and had been in a coma, totally unresponsive, for more than three months. Her biologic life was maintained by a feeding tube passed into the stomach via the nose, and by intravenous fluids. She had to be assisted in all her bodily functions.

She was in an eastern hospital at a cost of $180 per day, of which Medicare paid the greater part, but the family had to assume $50 daily. The family was eager to put an end to the situation and could see no sense in continuing life.

The physician in charge just could not bring himself to discontinue the maintenance treatments. He was quite amenable to the family's changing physicians or institutions, but the son could not find a physician who would consent to take the case. And so an elderly, completely comatose woman was kept alive. What is ironical is that the woman had told her family, some months prior to this stroke, that she was quite ready to die and that she hoped no one would force her to stay alive when her time came.

As the days passed with no change in the patient's condition, she was transferred to a room at the end of the hall. The room she vacated, close to the nursing station, could better be used for acutely ill patients whose progress could be monitored by the nursing staff. The care of Mrs. B was relegated to the newest and least experienced nurses' aides. Rarely did an RN look in on Mrs. B. What was the use? What was the need? There would be no change in her condition. The physician began to make fewer hospital visits, just sufficient to comply with the requirements of Medicare and the hospital's utilization review committee.

IN NURSING HOME

Mr. C, age 59 and alone in the world with no relatives, was a salesman for a small manufacturing company when he developed dysphagia (difficulty in swallowing). At first he ignored this problem, but after several months this six-foot man's weight dropped from his normal 180 pounds to a mere 138 pounds. He experienced pain when swallowing, began to regurgitate what little food he could force down, and developed a persistent hacking cough. Finally, he saw his internist, who, after radiographic examination and esophagoscopy diagnosed his condition as esophageal carcinoma.

Since Mr. C had a nonresectable tracheo-esophageal fistula (a hole between the trachea and the esophagus that could not be repaired surgically), a palliative bypass operation of the esophagus was performed. The patient, although weakened, after several days was able to eat and drink almost normally. By this time he was unable to return to work, and his meager savings had been depleted, forcing him to apply for Medicaid assistance through the hospital's social worker. Two weeks after the operation, he was transferred to a nursing home to live out his limited days.

He spent most of his time in his bed or a wheelchair. Few nursing personnel were available when he needed them. Sometimes he went without a bath for three or four consecutive days. Several times he could not attract the attention of an orderly to help him to the bathroom and sat in wet pajamas for hours before help arrived.

Mr. C had always prided himself on being somewhat intellectual, and he had read considerably before his illness struck. Now he had little desire to read, wiling away his days watching television or talking to his 80-year-old, senile roommate, who could not respond.

He complained of the stench of urine and feces throughout the facility; he complained of the boredom, the lack of attention, the loneliness of seldom being able to talk with another rational human being. The food was barely palatable to him; beer, liquor, and wine were not served to patients. He wished the window in his room would be cleaned occasionally so that he could at least look outdoors. And once he was settled into a wheelchair, he had great difficulty maneuvering without aid—not because he was too weak, but because the chair's wheel bearings needed replacement; six of the eight chairs he had used during his stay were in the same condition.

Thus Mr. C was destined to live out his remaining days, essentially alone, with virtually no intellectual stimulation, although his mind was alert. Even one of his few remaining enjoyments was denied him—that of eating good food and having an occasional highball.

IN HOSPICE

Mrs. D, a 28-year-old mother of five-year-old twin boys, was suffering from leukemia. Her hematologist, Dr. X, was unable to control the progression of the disease satisfactorily by means of chemotherapy. He informed the patient's husband that his wife was terminally ill and had a few weeks, at most, to live. Dr. X made arrangements for Mrs. D to be admitted to M Hospice.

Mrs. D's ambulance was met at the hospice's entrance by the head nurse and two orderlies, who welcomed Mrs. D and zipped her to her room in her own rolling bed. She was greeted by the hospice medical director and immediately put onto a chemotherapy regimen developed in consultation with her hematologist. Because she was in constant pain, a drug therapy program was immediately developed.

Her room was an airy, bright four-bed ward shared with three other women who had terminal illnesses. The nurses came in frequently to chat with the women, to offer encouragement, and to administer each of the patient's prescribed regimen medication. Volunteers brought flowers from the garden and books from the library, and spent hours with the four women, chatting, holding hands, listening, observing, offering suggestions, and running errands.

Mr. D frequently brought the twins to visit their mother. He brought her favorite rocking chair for her to use whenever she wanted to get out of bed and her favorite afghan for her to wear whenever she felt chilly. For the evening meals that they often shared, he brought cocktails and wine from home. Two or three times a week, Rover, the family dog, would also visit.

Her medication was administered every four hours, without fail; within the first 48 hours, she was free of pain. The medical director, the nurses, the housekeeping personnel, the chaplain, the social worker, the volunteers, and even the gardener collectively made her stay at M Hospice as pleasant as possible.

When Mrs. Y, her roommate, died, Mrs. D observed Mrs. Y's family and the hospice personnel arranged around the bed, grieving for the deceased. No curtains were drawn, no mystery surrounded the death. Mrs. Y had died, and the family and hospice grieved—a healthy phenomenon.

And when Mrs. D died three weeks later, she was content; she was peaceful. Her husband and her family knew that she had lived her last days in relative serenity, surrounded by people and things she loved. She had been surrounded by people who cared for her as an individual, as a fellow human being.

WHAT IS HOSPICE?

Hospice is not easy to define. It has been characterized as a caring community. It is a program for the terminally ill and their families. It is a philosophy of "providing an environment in which to die, but not of actively prolonging life or accelerating death."[4] Terry Miller, a nurses' aide at Hillhaven Hospice, Tucson, Arizona, calls hospice "a place to stop and rest before one's death. It is a place to do one's finishing up, to collect one's life together before saying goodbye to all with which one is familiar."[5] Another person has defined hospice as "a dream made from the nightmare called cancer; a place where dying people and their families are always considered as individuals with unique needs requiring unique health care personnel with everyone contributing his special gifts."[6]

Sister Teresa Marie, executive director of Hillhaven Hospice, puts it this way:

> No one is born alone. He is given life by another. No one lives alone; I learned who I am by seeing my reflection in others' eyes.

> Sometimes it is my turn to give, sometimes to receive. Giving and receiving—that is why Hospice is here. That is why we are here. We give what we have, and we give what we are; we want to give freely; we want to be among those "who deeply love" and "give love to all." We are already seeing that "more love returns." Let us remember that giving and receiving are not two sides of the ledger, but that both are simply coins of the realm, representing lasting riches. We will continue to make Hospice a treasure house.[7]

Douglas McKell, in a brochure describing hospice, defined it as follows:

> Hospice is not specifically a place, it is a concept of care. The purpose of hospice care is to improve the quality of a patient's and family's life by alleviating pain and recognizing that dying patients have special physical, emotional, social and spiritual needs. Hospice is dedicated to the concept of total family care. What the hospice concept of care offers is an environment for the family members to be involved in the process of a loved one dying.[8]

The St. Christopher's Hospice Annual Report for 1976–1977 indicated that "a hospice should be a more general term, as including continuing and palliative care units or teams and also those who prefer to simply call themselves a 'home.' On no account, however, should it mean merely 'custodial care.' "[9]

A preliminary definition of a hospice program of care was developed by the National Hospice Organization (NHO). It is presented here with the understanding that at this writing it is subject to further revision.

> Hospice is a medically directed, nurse coordinated program providing a continuum of home and inpatient care for the terminally ill patient and family. It employs an interdisciplinary team acting under the direction of an autonomous hospice administration. The program provides palliative and supportive care to meet the special needs arising out of the physical, emotional, spiritual, social and economic stresses which are experienced during the final stages of illness, and during dying and bereavement. This care is available 24 hours a day, seven days a week and is provided on the basis of need regardless of [ability] to pay. Such care of necessity requires careful record keeping for coordination of patient care as well as for use in education and research.[10]

The modern usage of the word *hospice* began in Britain in the middle of the nineteenth century with Mary Aikenhead, who founded the Irish Sisters of Charity. Since she considered death to be the beginning of the final journey, she naturally called her nursing home by the name of a resting place on a medieval pilgrimage to the Holy Land—a hospice.[11]

WHY HOSPICE?

As shown in the hypothetical cases of Mrs. B and Mr. C, the care of terminally ill patients in hospitals and nursing homes leaves a great deal to be desired. By contrast, the loving and compassionate care provided in a hospice comforts terminally ill patients as well as their families and eases the patients into death. All symptoms are controlled and the patient is prepared for death. Patient and family find that death can be beautiful though sorrowful. And the hospice staff will continue to care for the family for a time, usually six months to a year after the patient's death. As Richard Lamerton has written, "when cure is no longer the aim, the staff will use their skill to bring the patient comfort, treating each symptom as it arises."[12]*

QUALITY OF LIFE

Quality of life for the dying means maintaining *real* life as long as possible, ensuring that the patient is alert and comfortable, capable of enjoying family and surroundings, not desensitized by pain and anxiety.[13] Quality life includes observing the sunrise or sunset from an open window, listening to the birds sing, smelling the flowers, holding a baby, watching the joy of a child opening Christmas gifts, taking walks in the woods with loved ones (or, if the mood strikes, in solitude), traveling, reading, creating with mind and/or hands—enjoying the infinite activities of an active life.

Life is synonymous with fulfillment. If fulfillment is impossible, perhaps death is desirable and should be an available option after due consideration of all the factors concerned.[14] Medicine has a duty to relieve suffering and to preserve life, but it needs to re-examine its understanding of "life" as a merely physical phenomenon.[15]

---

*This and subsequent referenced citations from Richard Lamerton, *Care of the Dying*, reprinted by permission of Technomic Publishing Co., 265 Post Road West, Westport, Connecticut.

The idea that doctors and nurses must preserve life at all costs is an odd one and quite new. Never has this been their duty. The Hippocratic oath required a doctor to swear by the God of Health, not the God of Life. A doctor's concern should always be with the good health of the whole person, not with the longevity of the body.[16] With terminal patients, the aim should be not to prolong but to enrich the life that remains.[17]

> A patient should no more undergo aggressive treatment, which not only offers no hope of being effective, but which may isolate him from all true contact with those around him, than he should merely receive control of symptoms when the underlying cause is still treatable or has once again become so.[18]

As Dr. Eric Wilkes, medical director of St. Luke's Hospice in Sheffield, England has observed, it is "blasphemous" to hook dying people up to plumbing when what they really need is a friendly word, a hot cup of coffee, and some heroin.[19]

THE DIGNITY OF DEATH

Most people, if given the choice, would choose a dignified death. But what does this mean? The dignity of death is a concept difficult to define. It is a group of feelings, a sense (if one is conscious and aware at the time) that what is happening is appropriate, that it is a natural part of life.

Perhaps the dignity of death can be better defined by describing what it is not, rather than what it is. It is not being hooked up to a respirator, being kept artificially alive. It is not being tended, unable to care for our most basic needs and control our bodily functions. It is not being hopelessly senile, in agony, unable to function as a living, perceiving human being. As Joseph Fletcher puts it, "death control, like birth control, is a matter of human dignity."[20]

NOTES

1. Richard Lamerton, *Care of the Dying* (Westport, Connecticut: Technomic Publishing Co., 1976), p. 76.

2. Joan Craven and Florence S. Wald, "Hospice Care for Dying Patients," *American Journal of Nursing* 75 (October 1975): 1,816–22.

3. Robert A. Christensen, "When Each Extra Day Counts," *American Journal of Nursing* 77 (May 1977): 853.

4. *Hillhaven Hospice Medical Newsletter,* Hillhaven Hospice, Tucson, Arizona, 1, no. 1 (n.d.): 2.

5. Ibid., p. 3.

6. Ibid.

7. Ibid.

8. "Hospice Care—A New Concept for the Care of the Terminally Ill and Their Families," Workshop at UCLA Extension, Los Angeles, April 8–9, 1978.

9. St. Christopher's Hospice, "Annual Report, 1976–1977," p. 13.

10. National Hospice Organization, "Hospice Standards," 4th draft (Distributed to members of the National Hospice Organization Standard and Accreditation Committee, August 1, 1978), p. 2.

11. R. C. Lamerton, "The Need for Hospices," *Nursing Times* 71 (January 23, 1975): 155–7.

12. Lamerton, p. 35.

13. Linda Xiques, "Dying at Home," *Pacific Sun,* January 28–February 3, 1977.

14. G. A. Gresham, "A Time to be Born and a Time to Die," in *Euthanasia and the Right to Die,* ed. A. B. Downing (London: Peter Owen, 1969), pp. 148–51.

15. Joseph Fletcher, "The Patient's Right to Die," in *Euthanasia and the Right to Die,* ed. A. B. Downing (London: Peter Owen, 1969), pp. 61–70.

16. Lamerton, p. 81.

17. Dorothy H. Summers and Joan M. Young, *To Comfort Always* (London: St. Christopher's Hospice, (n.d.), p. 5.

18. Dr. Cicely Saunders, cited in Sandol Stoddard, *The Hospice Movement: A Better Way of Caring for the Dying* (Briarcliff Manor, N.Y.: Stein and Day, 1978), p. 95.

19. Michael Satchell, "How to Enjoy Life—Up to the Last Moment," *Parade,* October 16, 1977.

20. Fletcher, *loc. cit.*

Chapter 4

Attitudes Toward Death

Death is sometimes a punishment, sometimes a gift; to many it has come as a favor.

Seneca, *Hercules Oetaeus*

Death is a major life event. Death is a concern from the moment a person is born.[1] Parents and relatives ask themselves, either silently or aloud, "Will this child survive in the harsh world it is about to go into?" As we get older, these concerns about death are always with us, though probably, for most of us, they lie just below the surface of consciousness, brought to the surface only when triggered by some death-related incident.

Since, as Seneca proclaimed in *Hercules Furens*, "the hour which gives us life begins to take it away," we might then conclude that dying is a process that begins at birth and ends with death. Francis Bacon once wrote, "It is as natural to die as to be born."[2] Richard Lamerton tells us that "dying is normal—a healthy thing to do; everyone does it! Death is not an enemy to be swatted and parried to the last grim moment."[3]

THE CONSPIRACY OF SILENCE

While everyone agrees that death is natural, that dying is a part of living, it is not a part that we like to acknowledge. In fact, society seems to have collectively agreed not to discuss the subject. " 'The conspiracy of silence,' that tendency to avoid discussion of death at all cost, is not an isolated idiosyncrasy of attitude," claims Balfour Mount, "but a symptom of a deeper malaise which has developed to distort our perspective as we view death."[4]

Death and dying have been taboo topics in our culture for too many years. Norman Walter has called ours "one of the most death denying societies,"[5] while Lamerton contends that "our present-day conspiracy to ignore death looks like a community-sized act of cowardice."[6]

In contemporary American society, people never die; they "pass away." They are never dead, they are "departed"—as if death were only an extended vacation from the vicissitudes of life. When asked about the whereabouts of a patient who has died, unbeknown to the inquirer, hospital personnel reply that the patient has "left" or "gone," as if he or she had returned home or been transferred to another part of the hospital. In hospitalese, a patient "expires." Physicians, when reporting a death to a family offer the standard "I'm sorry, we did all that was humanly possible," as if the words "The patient has died" would be too great a shock. Then, too, family and friends, offering their condolences, respond, "We feel so bad" or "We know how you must feel," but they never mention about what.[7]

Many physicians fail to live up to their moral obligation by not admitting to their patients the terminal nature of their conditions. Physicians often feel that a terminal illness is a personal threat to their own abilities and are therefore unable to speak the truth.[8] Most people, however, are better equipped to bear the truth, no matter how devastating, than we give them credit for, and lack of candor can often lead to disastrous disruptions in personal relationships.[9]

People who are dying feel less isolated when they are able to share their feelings and thoughts about dying and death. Some patients can suffer more from an abrupt emotional isolation and unwitting rejection than from an illness per se. The opportunity to discuss their feelings may help subdue their fears of death.[10]

Despite our aversion to the subject, however, a new willingness to face the reality of death is developing, as evidenced by the approximately 40,000 courses, lectures, and seminars on death and dying that have been held in the United States in recent years.[11] It is estimated that in 1976 alone there were over 20,000 workshops, seminars, and lectures on the topic.[12] More is being written about death and dying than almost any other subject, apart from sex.[13]

FEAR OF DEATH

Many people have an inbred fear of death. As Krant has observed, "fear is frequently a property of the unknown." We are afraid of death because it is an unknown dimension. We do not know what we will exchange for life as we know it. "Be it nothingness, or a vague life form, or resurrection in our present body habitant, it is simply unknown." And adding to this fear is the fact that our modern society has made death an unacceptable topic of conversation, and therefore even more mysterious.[14]

People's fear of death can be broken down into three basic subfears: 1) the fear of physical pain and suffering, which are usually part of the dying process, 2) the fear of leaving one's loved ones behind, and 3) the fear of entering an unknown realm.[15] A study at the Royal Victoria Hospital revealed four more specific fears that terminally ill people commonly experience: 1) the fear of intolerable pain, 2) the fear of choking or suffocating, 3) the fear of deteriorating mentally and "losing control," and 4) the fear of being left alone at the moment of death.[16]

William Lamers, medical director of Hospice of Marin, spoke at the Third National Hospice Symposium of the fears and needs of terminally ill patients:

> The fears that people have are an indication of their needs. I've gone through some of our records and abstracted a number of fears presented to us.
>
> The fear of pain. The fear of suffering. The fear that this disease is meaningless. The fear of embarrassment. The fear of isolation. The fear of abandonment, of being sent to Coventry, [of not being associated with], of not being able to talk.
>
> The realistic fear, on the basis of the work of Glaser and Strauss, who wrote the book, *Awareness of Death,* which reflects the slowness with which nurses respond to calls from patients who have been declared incurable, as compared with those for whom there is still hope for cure.
>
> Fear of abandonment by physicians. The fear of death. The fear that what's happening to them is their punishment, and that they must endure it. The fear of financial drain, the loss of income, the cost of their illness. The fear of disfigurement. Loss of control. Fear of weakness. Fear of the unknown. The fear of being a burden on the family.
>
> The fear of being unable to care for oneself, or being unable to cope. The fear that others will be unable to cope.
>
> The fear of loss of function, loss of self-image, the fear of not having enough time. The thought of being better off dead. The fear that someone might, as the old Irish patients I saw used to say, be "given the black bottle."
>
> The fear of rejection because of their changed appearance. The fear of not being valued, of not being normal, of incontinence, of being a baby, of physical changes, of loss of sexual identity, of being dependent. The fear of recrimination, the "I told you so" kind of thing from angry family members.
>
> The fear of not being told the truth. In a recent poll it was found that 85%, roughly, of people wanted to be told the truth when they had a fatal illness.

> The fear of not being able to care for their children, of not having a full life, of deceit, misinformation, and broken promises.
>
> The lists of needs can also be expanded. Needs for openness. Openness with everyone. Need for honesty. The need for information about what's happening. The need of being able to participate in the decisions concerning one's own life and well-being.
>
> The need for open communication. The need to be valued just as I am. The need to be normal. Need to have relief from pain, for sleep, for understanding. To know one will not be abandoned by family and friends and physician.
>
> The need to be listened to. "Please hear me." The need to be cared for. The need to be loved. The need to be reassured that the family will get by after death has occurred. The need for continuing, integrated, good medical and nursing care. The need for family to be supportive, with respite to avoid burn-out.
>
> The need for care, comfort and answers to be available 24 hours a day, seven days a week. The need for peace and quiet. The need for control over visitors. The need for spiritual care and comfort. The need for some sort of hope, whether it be for cure, relief of pain, support, comfort, reassurance.
>
> Some of the questions that we frequently are asked are, "what's happening to me? What will happen to me? When will I die? How will I know? Who will help me? Will I be alone? Will I be aware of what's happening? Will I be in control? What will happen to my family?"[17]*

Yet despite these myriad fears, death, as Cicely Saunders, founder of London's St. Christopher's Hospice, succinctly wrote, "is not frightening when it is near or to the patient who is allowed to approach it in his own way."[18]

CULTURAL BELIEFS

Each culture has its own customs, traditions, and superstitions surrounding death. Different concepts of the soul and of the hereafter have produced different attitudes toward death and a wide variety of death customs. Many of these customs have been passed down through the centuries and have become part of our modern death traditions.

---

*From "The Needs of the Terminally Ill." Reprinted by permission of William M. Lamers, Jr., medical director, Hospice of Marin, Marin County, California.

Ancient cultures believed that the dead continued to live in a different form in the existing world. Hence, burial was seen as a way of preventing the return of the dead. In cases where there were particular reasons for concern, the dead were buried face down, and heavy boulders or tombstones were rolled on top. It may have been from such practices that the later use of a headstone or grave marker developed.[19] Interment was practiced as early as Paleolithic times. One possible reason for this is an idea that has apparently existed from very early times, that of planting the body in the earth like a seed for rebirth. Cave burials were also quite common in many societies.[20]

According to ancient beliefs, those thought to be virtuous were buried face up on an east-west axis with the head to the west. Most authorities believe that this was a carryover from the rites of early sun worshippers, borrowed and adapted by the Christians. According to early Christian tradition, final judgment will come from the east; thus, those who face the east can more easily rise.[21] A similar tradition existed in Ireland, where it was long a custom to remove the nails from the coffin just before lowering it into the grave so that the righteous might have no difficulty rising for the resurrection.[22]

A belief in the transmigration of the soul, or reincarnation, prevailed among many primitive peoples and in ancient Greece and Egypt. According to this belief, which is also part of the Hindu religion, after death the soul goes into the bodies of lower animals or the bodies of other human beings. The Greeks believed that the soul passes from one body to another until it is purified. It then returns to the dwelling place of its god. Brahmanic Hindus believe in the doctrine of *karma,* which decrees that what people do determines their destinies. If they live like animals, they will return to earth as animals. If they live fairly good lives, they will be reincarnated as human beings, rich or poor, beautiful or ugly, high or low on the social scale, depending upon the character of their previous lives. Eventually, the soul joins Brahman, the Universal Power.[23]

In the early centuries of the Roman civilization, the Romans' belief in life after death had an animistic nature. A person's soul, it was believed, although separated at death from the body, hovered around the place of burial for its continued happiness and required constant attention from the survivors—offerings of food and drink. If the offerings were stopped, the Romans thought that the soul would cease to be happy and might even become an evil spirit, bringing harm to those who had neglected the proper rites.[24]

Some cultures reserve particularly special treatment for their royalty and highly respected citizens. The ancient Scythians strangled their dead king's concubine, his cupbearer, his cook, his groom, his lackey, and his messenger and buried them with him, apparently to serve him in death. On the first anniversary of his death, they strangled 50 of the best of his attendants, with 50 of their most beautiful horses, to mark the occasion.[25] As do some societies in Africa today, the early Egyptians at times left the bodies of all except the more prominent members of the community, such as kings, governors, and nobles, to be devoured by wild animals or consumed by flesh-eating insects.[26]

Traditionally, old-time carpenters brushed together all of the sawdust and shavings accumulated from making a coffin and placed these scraps inside it. Superstition taught that if these bits of leftover wood were tracked into a house or carelessly shaken from clothing, they would endanger whomever they touched, and that person might become death's next victim.[27] Similarly, southern blacks in early America laid out their dead on a board and then placed a plate of salt and ashes beneath the board. The ashes were put there to absorb disease and at the graveside service were placed in the grave.[28]

Robert Jay Lifton reports that the Japanese have what may seem to us, because of our conflicts about death, a rather grotesque practice. He believes, however, that it has great value and beauty. After a cremation, close family members actually reach into a container with chopstick-like instruments and take out small pieces of the remains. They will then retain these pieces in their homes and will thus have some sense of connection with the deceased.[29] Although this may, at first, seem repugnant to us, it is not unlike the practice, common to both preliterate and modern societies, of bringing the deceased home for burial if the death occurred away from home. The United States government follows this practice with servicemen who have died overseas.[30]

A number of modern death customs can be traced back directly to age-old practices. The custom of funeral black is ancient. It originated from the belief that spirits, some of them ill-willed, hovered about a corpse. Black was worn to make the living inconspicuous and less apt to be troubled by evil spirits.[31] Possible continuations of primitive patterns can be seen in current practices such as the wearing of white gloves, an ancient sign of innocence, by pallbearers. Tolling of bells at a death was once seen as a means of driving demons away, as was the custom of lighting candles around the coffin.[32]

Another hoary death custom is inversion, inverting the body and associated artifacts after the death. Ancient mourners carried weapons upside down, returned from the burial ground in inverse order, walked backwards, turned clothing inside out, and, in some societies, even spoke backwards. Such practices seem to be related to the belief that the world of the dead is an inverted image of the living world, and so the mourners imitate the dead.[33] In 1963, millions of television viewers saw an example of an inversion when the riderless horse with boots backward in the stirrups pranced in President John F. Kennedy's funeral cortege.

Death as Reward

Rather than a vast unknown to be feared, a region populated by ill-willed spirits bent on haunting the living, or a strange, inverted world, the hereafter is viewed by many as a place for collecting one's reward. Death is also seen as a means of obtaining rewards for others as well as for oneself. Vernon offers several examples.

> Human sacrifice has been used by many in an effort to secure supernatural rewards or blessings. The Timpanagos Myths specify, for instance, that a certain type of maiden had to be sacrificed in order for her tribe to be assured of supernatural blessings. Religious convictions about the hereafter may facilitate death as they appeared to do for the early Christian martyrs who wanted to realize their heavenly reward earlier, . . . by laying down their lives for the faith. Their numbers became so large and their provocations of the civil authorities to impose the death penalties became so extensive that they contributed to the development of the present strictures in the Roman Catholic church against suicides.[34]

Many ancient Mayas committed suicide when they were depressed or even slightly annoyed, in the belief that suicides had a favored place in heaven under the protection of Ixtab, the goddess with the rope around her neck. World War II Japanese kamikaze pilots believed that their glorious self-sacrifice in battle would bring them spiritual rewards.[35] And, just as the Timpanagos maiden was sacrificed to ensure supernatural blessings for her people, in a modern-day variation of this practice some people commit suicide to provide insurance money for their families.

In his classic 1962 work *The Other America: Poverty in the United States,* Michael Harrington observed that at that time there were a disproportionate number of funeral parlors in this country's inner-city ghettos and that undertakers were among the most respected members of the black middle class. Death-benefit plans were common among black lodges and fraternal orders. For the poor, a funeral is a moment of style and status, one of life's few opportunities for luxury.[36]

Modern Death Denial

Although in most cultures death is not an event that is looked forward to, the death denial so characteristic of our modern society, particularly American society, was not always so strong. In the turn-of-the-century rural farm society, each farm unit was multigenerational; grandparents were not sent off to nursing homes but remained with the family. Few persons were born or died in hospitals. The children witnessed death, either of animals slaughtered for food, or of family members who died from accidents, illness, or old age. Children were not protected or sheltered from death.[37]

A death in the family was a shared event, with neighbors and grandchildren coming to pay their last respects. Death was accepted as a part of life. It happened naturally, every day, and was seen in the context of nature with its cycles of life and death.[38]

Pattison has written that "the taboos about death have been so strong that people have suggested it is harmful for children to see corpses and attend funerals."[39] Eissler has suggested that we should practice orthonasia; that is, we should teach children about death as part of life, so that they will develop healthy attitudes toward death and be adequately prepared to deal with death in their own lives.[40]

Phillipe Ariés, in an article about American funerals, reports that the practice of embalming, although characteristic of the American way of death, is almost unknown in Europe.[41] It is yet another phenomenon of our death-denying society; with the aid of embalming fluid, putty, cotton, and cosmetics, the deceased is given the appearance of life, of merely being asleep. The American funeral industry has perpetuated this practice to the point where survivors now expect and even demand to see the deceased in a state of pleasant repose, almost as if they refuse to accept the fact of death. Rozovsky claims that "throughout history man has been unable to disassociate the dead physical frame of a deceased person from the person of the deceased."[42]

Ariés, in writing of the role of the undertaker, argues that "mourning is no longer a necessary period imposed by society; it has become a *morbid state* which must be treated, shortened, erased by the 'doctor of grief'."[43] The undertaker has gone through a metamorphosis, beginning as a mortician and progressing to undertaker, then to funeral director, and now to what Ariés calls the "doctor of grief."

THEOLOGICAL VIEWS

The idea of death is fraught with horror. There has always existed a vague hope that it may be, if not explained, at least explained away, made unreal, denied. It was from humanity's efforts to adjust to the facts of death, to reduce the threat of death, that religion developed.[44]

Although early Christian martyrs died fearlessly in eager anticipation of eternal bliss, Christianity has, on the whole, used its vast influence to make people dread death. Some members of the clergy today use the threat of death to instill fear. A young girl dying of cancer was troubled because her clergyman had told her that she would never get to heaven because she "did not love God more than anyone else in the world," since he had overheard her telling her brother that she loved Mommy and Daddy more than anyone in the world.[45] Most Christians, however, consider a young child as being in a condition of purity. No rites or rituals, such as baptism, are necessary to ensure the direct return of the child to God, from whom it came.

Not all religions hold the threat of death as punishment over their followers' heads. In Buddhism, for example, the emphasis is not on good and evil, reward and punishment, repentance and forgiveness, but on enlightenment, on transcending all thought, anxiety, and desire. This difference in Buddhist and Christian attitudes is embodied in the stories of the deaths of Buddha and Christ. Buddha's serene death represents an outright antithesis to Christ's dreadful death.[46]

Because of the solemnity of the occasion, all religions demand that those ministering to the dying shall create as peaceful an atmosphere as possible. After the death, they all agree that the body must be treated with respect and gentleness.[47] The Roman Catholic church demands that not only the human body, but any part of the human body be accorded the utmost respect. Jewish religious law forbids the mutilation of the human body in any way whatsoever. Therefore, autopsies, dissections, and removal of parts are against religious law.[48] Today, when an Orthodox Jew must undergo an amputation, the limb is accorded full burial rights, as if the entire body were represented by the severed part.

The traditional Roman Catholic understanding of the moment of real death has been based on the time of departure of the soul from the body.[49] Lamerton claims that in the moment of death the person departs, leaving the body behind. Death is therefore a change of form. A prevalent belief is that a soul survives, in some other form. Eastern belief holds that the soul returns to manifest itself again in a new body.[50]

Finally, the twelfth-century Judaic Code of Maimonides (the Book of Judges, Law of Mourning, 4:5) lays down rules for caring for the dying that are considerably different from our modern rules.

> One who is in a dying condition is regarded as a living person in all respects. It is not permitted to bind his jaws, to stop up the

> organs of the lower extremities, or to place metallic or cooling vessels upon his navel in order to prevent swelling. He is not to be rubbed or washed, nor is sand or salt to be put upon him until he expires. He who touches him is guilty of shedding blood. To what may he be compared? To a flickering flame, which is extinguished as soon as one touches it. Whoever closes the eyes of the dying while the soul is about to depart is shedding blood. One should wait a while, perhaps he is only in a swoon.[51]

HEALTH PROFESSIONALS' VIEWS

A competent physician spends sleepless nights trying to decide how to tell a cheerful, alert octogenarian that her illness is terminal. A nurse in a geriatric hospital explains that she never upsets patients by telling them of the death of a close friend or wardmate. They are thus left to determine by themselves the significance of the empty bed. A young internist abruptly and coldly informs an elderly patient that she will be dead of cancer within three months. Although she actually lived for six months, the intern had achieved his real goal—to remove her impending death from his consciousness. A nursing home aide tells her friend, "Right after work, I go home, take a stiff shot, and forget about that depressing place until I show up in the morning."[52]

The topic of death is, as Edwin Shneidman has said, "an especially unpleasant one for medical personnel."[53] If the notion of death is distressing to patients and to their families, it is similarly distressing to physicians. For them it may represent technical failure, human and medical inadequacy, or simply the loss of a patient and friend.[54] A contrasting view is expressed by Richard Lamerton, who claims, "A man's death does not represent a humiliating defeat of medicine, but is the logical conclusion of life. To die well is a great achievement, a very positive step which makes a man so much the greater, so much more completely a man."[55]

A supervisory nurse, Eileen Strauss, expressed her concerns about medical professionals' conflicting attitudes about death.

> Doctors can very easily intellectually make a decision about the terminal patient. They will write an order for us, "Do not resuscitate." But if the patient dies when the doctor is on the ward, he immediately goes over and starts life-saving measures. It seems as though he is willing to write the order as long as I, if I am there, make the decision. I don't do anything. But if he is there, he himself cannot cope with the fact of not doing something to save the patient.[56]

Strauss added, "I resent the fact that in many cases the doctor does not act positively in a negative fashion, but expects me to do so. . . . I think that the education of doctors from medical school onward has to change in some ways."[57]

In working with the dying, health professionals must work through their own reactions to death and dying so that they can recognize and respect those same reactions in their patients and their families. They must be able to deal with the situation in a personal and professional capacity.[58]

Humanity and sensitivity are especially necessary qualities for people who provide care for terminally ill patients;[59] yet interns have been overheard in terminal wards of hospitals to say, with defensive gallows-humor, that they have to "go water the vegetables."[60]

On one occasion, a nurse at the Royal Victoria Hospital, Montreal, after being asked for assistance by a terminally ill patient, angrily complained, "Why doesn't she just die and leave us alone!"[61]

Children, it seems, fare somewhat better, often receiving more personal and higher-quality or more extensive care. Glaser and Strauss suggest that this is because, in American society, a high value is placed on having a full life. The loss of a child, who has not had the chance to live a full life, is therefore viewed as a greater loss than that of an adult or an aged individual.[62]

Cicely Saunders, in writing specifically about the terminal cancer patient, speaks of the need for both the doctor and the patient to take a positive, accepting approach to the coming death.

> Some will find it shocking that we should speak of the accepting or even preparing for death and will think that both patient and doctor should believe in treatment and fight for life right up to the end. They may question how anyone should be satisfied with what sounds such a negative role. To talk of accepting death when its approach has become inevitable is not mere resignation on the part of the patient nor defeatism or neglect on the part of the doctor. Certainly they will take no steps to hasten its coming, but for both of them it is the very opposite of doing nothing. The patient may well achieve more in this part of his life than in any other, making of it a real reconciliation and fulfillment.[63]

THE STAGES OF DYING

In 1965, four theological students approached Elisabeth Kubler-Ross, one of the modern authorities on death and dying, for assistance in writing a class paper on the greatest crisis people had to face. The four had selected death as their topic, but the question arose, How do you perform research on dying when the data are practically impossible to obtain, when you cannot verify your data or set up experiments? They decided to ask terminally ill patients to be their teachers. They would observe critically ill patients, study their responses and needs, evaluate the reactions of people around them, and get as close to the dying as they would allow. Thus were born the seminars on death and dying for which Kubler-Ross is famous.[64]

Kubler-Ross is also known for her pioneering work in identifying the five stages of dying: 1) denial and isolation, 2) anger, 3) bargaining, 4) depression, and 5) acceptance.[65] Of course, not every dying person proceeds neatly through all five stages, but one or more stages can usually be distinguished. Kubler-Ross says that these five stages are only guidelines and should not be considered definite stages through which all people go.[66]

One person who takes issue with the concept of distinct, identifiable stages of dying is Edwin Shneidman. "Rather than the five definite stages [of Kubler-Ross]," Shneidman writes, "my experience leads me to posit a hive of affect, in which there is a constant coming and going." He has observed a constant interplay between disbelief and hope, a "waxing and waning of anguish, terror, acquiescence and surrender, rage and envy, disinterest and ennui, pretense, taunting and daring, and even yearning for death—all these in the context of bewilderment and pain."[67]

Feifel contends that we can accept a delineation of sequential stages of dying as a guide but that these stages are not "inexorable hoops through which most dying patients inevitably pass." He has found that these presumed stages can coexist, that the purported sequences can be reversed or even skipped. Feifel claims that some members of the helping professions, however, almost force dying patients to jump through those inferred hoops.[68]

SOCIAL DEATH

Sudnow describes social death as a phenomenon incorporating the process of "mutual disengagement and rejection by which . . . the human being as a member of society seems prone to take his leave from the land of the living."[69] A tentative distinction can be made between *clinical death* (the appearance of "death signs" upon physical examination), *biological death* (the cessation of cellular activity), and a third category, *social death,* which is that point at which a dying person is treated essentially as a corpse, though perhaps still "clinically" and "biologically" alive—not an uncommon phenomenon.[70]

At one county hospital, patients who were admitted at death's door—with extremely low blood pressure, erratic heartbeats, and nonpalpable or weak pulse rates—were frequently left on their litters and wheeled into a laboratory or large supply room. In such a case, a nurse explained, they did not want to use a bed and have to clean the room afterward. Since the patient would soon die, there was no need to assign a room. In several cases, patients were left throughout the night and died in the supply room. Those who were still alive in the morning, nurses quickly assigned to beds, before the arrival of physicians or relatives. In effect, a patient admitted in critical condition was treated as a corpse by night and a patient by day.[71]

A man was admitted to a hospital emergency department with a sudden perforation of a duodenal ulcer. He was operated upon, and, for six days, remained in critical condition. His wife was informed that his chances of survival were poor, whereupon she stopped her visits to the hospital. After two weeks the man's condition improved markedly, and he was discharged in ambulatory condition. The next day, he was re-admitted to the hospital with a severe coronary. Before he died he related his experience upon returning home. His wife had removed all of his clothing and personal effects from the house and had made preliminary arrangements for his burial (she had written a letter, which he discovered on his bureau, requesting a brochure on funeral rates). She no longer wore his wedding ring and was found with another man, no doubt quite shocked at her husband's return. He reported that he left the house, began to drink heavily, and had a heart attack.[72]

A nurse on duty with a dying woman was observed spending some two or three minutes trying to close the woman's eyelids. This involved slowly but somewhat forcefully pushing the two lids together to get them to adhere in a closed position. After several unsuccessful moments, she managed to get them to stay shut and said, with a sigh of accomplishment, "Now they're right." When questioned about what she had been doing, she said that a patient's eyelids are always closed after death, so that the body will resemble a sleeping person. She explained that since, after death, it is more difficult to close the eyelids, especially after the muscles have begun to tighten, she always tried to close them before death, while they are still easily manipulated.[73]

Once patients have been declared incurable, those not accustomed to treating the dying tend to forget them, to withdraw quickly and leave them alone. Patients sense a deep abyss of desolation and loneliness; they become depressed and introverted. They may exhibit resentment and aggression, or just an overwhelming hopelessness. They sleep most of the time, withdrawing from the world "into a dark and haunted cavern of dreams and drifting imaginings. This is real suffering."[74]

Patients must not feel rejected by those they have trusted. Almost all patients express fear that their conditions will make them so unacceptable to those around them that they will be abandoned.[75] From terminally ill patients in acute-care general hospitals are often heard statements such as, "I don't belong here. I'm not getting any better. I must be a disappointment to my doctors and everybody. I'm not getting well like I'm supposed to. Why don't they just take me out and shoot me?" Feeling unwanted, like a misfit, sensing that you are a disappointment to others, is no way to approach the end of life.[76]

In an interview, the National Cancer Institute's Larry Burke commented, "Historically, the terminally ill have died in an ignoble way . . . because when you become terminally ill, you're lumped in with custodial care patients, minimal physical needs are provided for, and no psychological needs [are attended to] at all. This system says: 'the medical men have given up on you, we're going to withdraw from you.' "[77] The hospice attempts to minimize the phenomenon of social death, substituting care and attention for the abandonment and isolation so common in the hospital setting.

GRIEF AND BEREAVEMENT

Mourning is our natural way of coping with loss. The effort involved in grieving has been divided into "worry work" before the loved person dies and "grief work" afterwards.[78] Grief is the emotion that is involved in the work of mourning, whereby people seek to disengage themselves from demanding relationships that have existed and to reinvest their emotional capital in new and productive directions for their future health and welfare.[79]

Part of the care of the dying is care of the bereaved; they are two sides of the same coin. It is important to understand that grief begins from the moment a member of the family is told that the patient will not recover.[80]

> A terminal illness is not like an acute illness. In an acute illness, although the short term stress may be great, the long term hope and anticipation is that full family function will be restored and life will go on as it did before. In a terminal illness every member of the family is pulled in and affected by the illness. Adjustments to living without the patient begin before death, as functions previously fulfilled by the patient have to be taken over by other

> members of the family. We must aim to involve the family from the beginning.[81]

Any consideration of the patient's needs is incomplete without attention to the family's needs.

> While it may seem, at first glance, that it is the patient who faces the greatest ordeal in the context of the terminal setting, this is often not the case. For when we consider the magnitude of the emotional crisis faced by the family, their unresolved psychological and religious problems, their conflicts of identification with the dying person, their prospective loss of one who has meant so much, we come to realize that the terminal setting can be more disruptive and frustrating for those who live than for the person who dies. That this is true is all too evident from the fact that many families find themselves torn apart, both physically and spiritually, by their confrontation with death.[82]

Dr. Charles Bachmann describes "anticipatory grief reaction," especially in long-term terminal cases: "the relatives may so much anticipate the death of the father or mother . . . that in their minds, they already buried him or her before he actually dies. They go through the usual grief process before death, and observers may report a tearless grief reaction."[83]

Adult mourners pass through three stages: a short period of shock, usually lasting between the occurrence of death and the disposal of the body; a period of intense mourning, accompanied by the withdrawal of much attention and affect from the external world and by such physiological changes as disturbed and restless sleep, often with vivid dreams, loss of appetite, and loss of weight; and a final period of re-established physical homeostasis—sleep and weight again stabilized and interest again directed outward.[84]

Grieving begins before death occurs and continues after death. Patient, family, friends, and those who give care all experience the sorrow to some degree; they all need comfort. The bereaved are more vulnerable to physical and psychological disease; care for the survivors, therefore, is as legitimate a concern of health professionals as preventive medicine. It begins while caring for the patient and is needed until the survivors can cope for themselves, or until other resources such as mental health services, the family physician, other relatives, or clergy can provide the help still needed.[85]

Normal grief generally proceeds through a series of predictable stages, though all mourners will work through their own variation of the problem.

> At first for a few days, only occasionally for more than a week, the person behaves almost as if nothing has happened. He handles day to day affairs like an automaton, feeling numb and empty. . . . After this numbness the pangs of grief begin. . . . Illusions of the presence of the dead person are common and normal, and may continue to occur at intervals for a decade or so. . . . The pangs of grief gradually give way to depression and despair as the person unlearns the habits he has woven around the relationship with the deceased. . . . One particularly difficult day is the first anniversary of the death. A visit from a friend, clergyman, or doctor is then welcomed, and some hospices send a postcard with an offer of help if needed. After two years or so, it may eventually be appropriate to point out to a person who is still grieving that their duty to the dead is now done and grieving has gone on long enough.[86]

One of the most effective ways to cope with grief is to understand that the feelings of guilt, resentment, of not having done enough, desertion, deprivation, anger, fear, and countless others are shared by almost all who grieve. Since death is not a subject for casual conversation, however, two people in a family may be grieving for the same person and experiencing almost identical emotional reactions, but because they do not feel free to bare these emotions completely, they may assume that their own reactions are abnormal.[87]

The act of grieving, in itself, has a definite therapeutic quality. The family of the deceased has an opportunity not only to think through the loss of the one they loved, but also to recollect their thoughts and to begin life anew with a deeper and more profound understanding of its meaning, both for the present and the future.[88]

One final thought from Richard Lamerton: "It is important to say goodbye. A conspiracy of silence will worsen the dying person's sense of isolation and stores up later emotional problems for the bereaved."[89]

NOTES

1. E. Mansell Pattison, *The Experience of Dying* (Englewood Cliffs, New Jersey: Prentice-Hall, 1977), p. 2.

2. Francis Bacon, "Of Death," *Essaies of Sir Francis Bacon* (London: John Beale, 1612).

3. Richard Lamerton, *Care of the Dying* (Westport, Connecticut: Technomic Publishing Co., 1976), p. 79.

4. Balfour Mount, "Death—A Part of Life?" *Crux* 11, no. 3 (1973–1974): 3–6.

5. Norman T. Walter, "The Coming of Death in America: Concepts in Transition," mimeographed, July 15, 1976, p. 5.
6. Lamerton, p. 114.
7. Carl G. Carlozzi, *Death and Contemporary Man: The Crisis of Terminal Illness* (Grand Rapids: William B. Eerdmans Publishing Co., 1968), pp. 24–5.
8. Ibid., p. 62.
9. Frederic P. Herter, "The Right To Die in Dignity," *Death and Bereavement,* ed. Austin H. Kutscher (Springfield, Illinois: Charles C Thomas, 1969), pp. 14–19.
10. Herman Feifel, "Death," in *Taboo Topics,* ed. Norman L. Faberow (New York: Atherton Press, 1963), p. 17.
11. D. G. McCarthy, "Should Catholic Hospitals Sponsor Hospices?" *Hospital Progress* 57 (December 1976): 61–5.
12. Elisabeth Kubler-Ross, "Living with Dying," Speech sponsored by Power Within, Lobero Theater, Santa Barbara, California, October 4, 1977.
13. Lorne E. Rozovsky, "Death, Dead Bodies and the Law," *Canadian Hospital,* July 1970, pp. 52–5.
14. Melvin J. Krant, *Dying and Dignity: The Meaning and Control of a Personal Death* (Springfield, Illinois: Charles C Thomas, 1974), p. 29.
15. Carlozzi, pp. 19–21.
16. *Palliative Care Service: October 1976 Report* (Montreal: Royal Victoria Hospital, McGill University, 1976), p. 354.
17. William M. Lamers, Jr., "The Needs of the Terminally Ill and Those Close to Them" (Paper delivered at *The "How to" of Hospice Care,* Third National Symposium, Dominican College Campus, San Rafael, California, May 26–28, 1977), pp. 7–8.
18. Cicely Saunders, "The Need for In-Patient Care for the Patient with Terminal Cancer," *Middlesex Hospital Journal* 72 (February, 1973).
19. Glenn M. Vernon, *Sociology of Death* (New York: Ronald Press, 1970), p. 217.
20. A. M. Hocart, "Death Customs," *Encyclopedia of the Social Sciences,* ed. Seligman and Johnson (New York: MacMillan, 1931).
21. Vernon, p. 217.
22. Vern L. Bullough, "The Banal and Costly Funeral," *The Humanist* 4 (1960): 213–18.
23. Wilson D. Wallis, "Transmigration of the Soul," *World Book Encyclopedia,* 1967.
24. William G. Sumner and Albert Keller, *The Science of Society* (New Haven: Yale University Press, 1927), p. 11.
25. Milton Mayer, "On Death," *The Great Ideas Today, 1965,* ed. Robert M. Hutchins and Mortimer Adler (Chicago: Encyclopedia Britannica, Inc., 1965), pp. 107–64.
26. E. A. Wallis Budge, *The Book of the Dead* (New Hyde Park, New York: University Books, 1960), p. 3.
27. Margaret M. Coffin, *Death in Early America* (New York: Thomas Nelson, 1976), pp. 102–3.
28. Ibid., p. 79.
29. "We Who Stand at the Border of Life and Death" (Interview with Robert Jay Lifton), *Prism* 3 (June 1975): 46–49, ff.
30. Vernon, p. 225.
31. Coffin, p. 196.

32. Bullough, loc. cit.
33. Hocart, loc. cit.
34. Vernon, p. 42.
35. Ibid., pp. 40–2.
36. Michael Harrington, *The Other America: Poverty in the U.S.* (Baltimore: Penguin Books, 1963), pp. 69–70.
37. Krant, pp. 7–8.
38. Mount, loc. cit.
39. E. Mansell Pattison, ed. *The Experience of Dying* (Englewood Cliffs, New Jersey: Prentice-Hall, 1977), p. 28.
40. Kurt R. Eissler, *The Psychiatrist and the Dying Patient* (New York: International Universities Press, 1955).
41. Phillipe Ariés, "A Moment That Has Lost Its Meaning," *Prism* 3 (June 1975): 27–9, ff.
42. Rozovsky, loc. cit.
43. Ariés, loc. cit.
44. Vernon, p. 58.
45. Cited by Kubler-Ross, "Living with Dying."
46. Walter Kaufmann, "Existentialism and Death," *The Meaning of Death,* ed. Herman Feifel (New York: McGraw Hill Book Co., 1959), pp. 39–63.
47. Lamerton, p. 139.
48. Rozovsky, loc. cit.
49. Frank Veith et al., "Brain Death: I. A Status Report of Medical and Ethical Considerations," *JAMA* 238 (October 10, 1977): 1,651–5.
50. Lamerton, p. 145.
51. Cited in Fred Rosner, *Studies in Torah Judaism: Modern Medicine and Jewish Law* (New York: Yeshiva University, 1972), p. 118.
52. Richard A. Kalish, "The Aged and the Dying Process: The Inevitable Decisions," *Journal of Social Issues* 21 (1965): 87–96.
53. Edwin Shneidman, *Deaths of Man* (Baltimore: Penguin Books, 1974), p. 38.
54. F. E. Lucente, "Thanatology: A Study of 100 Deaths," *Transactions of American Academy of Ophthalmology and Otolaryngology* 76 (March-April, 1972): 334–9.
55. Lamerton, p. 76.
56. Eileen Strauss, in *Dilemmas of Euthanasia: Excerpts from Papers and Discussion at the 4th Euthanasia Conference* (New York: The Euthanasia Educational Council, 1971), p. 38.
57. Ibid.
58. *Palliative Care Service,* p. 85.
59. Emily Freidman, "California Hospitals Design Natural Death Act Procedures," *Hospitals* 51 (November 16, 1977): 62–5.
60. Joseph Fletcher, "The Patient's Right to Die," *Euthanasia and the Right To Die,* ed. A. B. Downing (London: Peter Owen, 1969), pp. 61–70.
61. *Palliative Care Service,* p. 156.
62. Barney Glaser and Anselm Strauss, "The Social Loss of Dying Patients," *American Journal of Nursing* 63 (January 1964): 119–21.
63. Saunders, "The Need for In-Patient Care."
64. Elisabeth Kubler-Ross, *On Death and Dying* (New York: MacMillan, 1969), p. 19.

65. Ibid., pp. 34–121.

66. Kubler-Ross, "Living with Dying."

67. Shneidman, p. 7.

68. Herman Feifel, "Death and Dying in Modern America," *Death Education* 1 (Spring 1977): 5–14.

69. David Sudnow, "Dying in a Public Hospital," *The Dying Patient,* ed. Orville G. Brim, Jr., et al. (New York: Russell Sage Foundation, 1970), pp. 191–208.

70. David Sudnow, *Passing On: The Social Organization of Dying* (Englewood Cliffs, N.J.: Prentice-Hall, 1967), p. 74.

71. Sudnow, "Dying in a Public Hospital," loc. cit.

72. Sudnow, *Passing on,* p. 77.

73. Ibid., p. 74.

74. Lamerton, p. 55.

75. Glen W. Davidson, *Living with Dying* (Minneapolis: Augsberg Publishing House, 1975), p. 23.

76. Edward F. Dobihal, Jr., "Talk or Terminal Care?" *Connecticut Medicine* 38 (July 1974): 364–7.

77. Alsofrom, J., "Hospice Way of Dying—At Home with Friends and Family." *American Medical News* 20 (February 21, 1977): 7–9.

78. Lamerton, p. 125.

79. Edgar Jackson, *Understanding Grief* (Nashville: Abingden, 1957), p. 18.

80. Lamerton, p. 124.

81. Sylvia Lack, "Philosophy and Organization of a Hospice Program," unpublished paper, n.d.

82. Carlozzi, p. 41.

83. Charles C. Bachmann, *Ministering to the Grief Sufferer* (Englewood Cliffs, N.J.: Prentice-Hall, 1964), pp. 23–4.

84. Geoffrey Gorer, *Death, Grief, and Mourning in Contemporary Britain* (London: The Cresset Press, 1965), p. 112.

85. Joan Craven and Florence S. Wald, "Hospice Care for Dying Patients," *American Journal of Nursing* 75 (October 1975): 1,816–22.

86. Lamerton, pp. 127–31.

87. Glenn Mosely, "Guilt," in *Death and Bereavement,* ed. Austin H. Kutscher (Springfield, Illinois: Charles C Thomas, 1969), pp. 210–11.

88. Carlozzi, p. 49.

89. Lamerton, p. 20.

Chapter 5
The Right To Die

Tir'd with all these, for restful death I cry
Shakespeare, *Sonnet LXVI*

The right to die with dignity should be recognized as a basic human right.[1] Death is a blessing when it ends a life wracked with suffering and stripped of its meaning. The prolongation of suffering is not a compassionate act.[2] By maintaining an essentially dead person on life support systems for no reason, our economic and social resources are irresponsibly squandered. Such a practice places an unnecessary financial burden on society and an additional emotional burden on the person's family.[3]

The Legislative Newsletter of the Society for the Right to Die reported that a 1977 Lou Harris poll indicated that 71 percent of Americans believe that "a patient with a terminal disease ought to be able to tell his doctor to let him die rather than to extend his life when no cure is in sight." This represents a change in public attitude from 1973, when 62 percent felt the same way.[4]

EUTHANASIA

Euthanasia is the practice of painlessly putting to death those who have incurable, painful, or distressing diseases or handicaps. The word comes from the Greek *eu,* meaning "good," and *thanatos,* meaning "death,"—hence, a good or easy death.

The Nazis believed in eugenics, the scientific improvement of hereditary racial qualities. They considered the slaughtering of six million healthy, intelligent, capable human beings, because they were Jewish,

---

The issue of the right to die, which includes the issue of euthanasia, is an exceptionally emotional and volatile one. The reader is cautioned not to equate euthanasia with the hospice program of care for patients and their families. Those not familiar with hospices, however, should be permitted to determine where euthanasia fits into the overall perspective of death and dying.

"mercy killings" that were a necessary part of their racial "improvement" program. Euthanasia, or "mercy killing," has therefore been associated with the Nazi philosophy. Euthanasia has a negative connotation in the minds of many people also because there are those who advocate its use for the purpose of ridding society of the "unfit" and those who are burdens on society, such as the aged, habitual criminals, and people with incurable illnesses.[5]

Direct, Indirect, and Voluntary Euthanasia

Joseph Fletcher has used the terms *dysthanasia* and *antidysthanasia* in describing the physician's role.[6] The word *dysthanasia* is derived from the Greek prefix *dys* meaning "bad," and *thanatos* meaning "death,"—the opposite of euthanasia. Dysthanasia is the useless prolongation of life, which only increases suffering.[7] Antidysthanasia, then, is synonymous with indirect euthanasia (sometimes referred to as passive or negative euthanasia), which is inducing death by not giving help or treatment. Direct euthanasia (sometimes referred to as active or positive euthanasia) is inducing death by doing or giving something, for example, an intravenous injection[8] (see Table 5-1). "A deliberate act of omission, when death is the goal or purpose or end sought," said Joseph Fletcher, "is morally

Table 5-1 Classifications of Euthanasia

Dysthanasia (bad death)	Euthanasia (easy or good death)		
	Passive or Negative Euthanasia (antidysthanasia)	Active or Positive Euthanasia	
		Indirect	Direct
Prolongation of suffering. Use of extraordinary means or "heroic" efforts to prolong life uselessly.	Desisting from or discontinuing useless prolongation. An act of omission which permits natural death to occur.	Indirectly causing death by use of drugs to relieve pain but which clearly hasten death.	Deliberately inducing death in order to terminate hopeless suffering or a meaningless existence.

Source: Reprinted by permission of the publisher from O. Ruth Russell, *Freedom to Die* (New York: Human Sciences Press, 1975), p. 23. © 1975 by Human Sciences Press, 72 Fifth Ave., New York, New York 10011.

the same, no better nor worse in the forum of conscience than a deliberate act of commission." He added, "Not to do anything is a decision to act."[9]

When patients with terminal illnesses request, or even plead, for their lives to be ended because of the uselessness, hopelessness, and agony of enduring prolongation of life by mechanical support systems, this act may be known as voluntary euthanasia. Glanville Williams claims that the argument in favor of voluntary euthanasia is quite simple and is an application of two values that are widely recognized. The first value is the prevention of cruelty. Those who plead for the legislation of euthanasia think that it is cruel to allow human beings to linger for months in the last stages of agony, weakness, and decay and to refuse them their demand for merciful release. The second value is that of liberty. Williams states that the criminal law should not be involved to repress conduct unless this is demonstrably necessary on social grounds. What social interest, he questions, is served by preventing the sufferer from choosing to accelerate death by a few months? What positive social value does that life still possess that the dying person is to be retained in it by the terrors of the criminal law?[10] Emil Freireich, however, presented an opposing viewpoint in a discussion at the Seventh Annual Euthanasia Conference: "The concept that you can be kind by doing murder offends my concepts of morality. It is the basic communist doctrine of any evil for an ultimate good."[11]

Barrington contends that the prolonged period of dying that is suffered by so many incurable patients who are kept alive to be slowly killed by their disease is not a natural process.[12]

> The sufferings of animals (other than man) are heart-rending enough, but a dying process spread over weeks, months, or years seems to be one form of suffering that animals are normally spared. When severe illness strikes them, they tend to stop eating, sleep and die. The whole weight of Western society forces attention on the natural right to live, but throws a blanket of silence over the natural right to die.[13]

Too, the family's suffering must be considered. There is nothing more tragic than the disruption of happy and productive family life by a prolonged terminal illness, and needless prolongation turns what might have been a happy and respectful memory into a nightmare and a horror.[14]

The Medical View

The medical view of euthanasia is expressed in the American Medical Association guidelines adopted in 1973.

> The intentional termination of the life of one human being by another—mercy killing—is contrary to that for which the medical profession stands and is contrary to the policy of the American Medical Association. The cessation of the employment of extraordinary means to prolong the life of the body when there is irrefutable evidence that biological death is imminent is the decision of the patient and/or his immediate family. The advice and judgment of the physician should be freely available to the patient and/or his immediate family.[15]

In 1887, William Munk wrote of euthanasia, not in the sense of mercy killing, but in the sense of good death—making patients comfortable in their last days or hours. He claimed that the fewer the drugs and the less medicine we can do with in the treatment of the dying, the better. "In very many cases there is no need of medicines of any kind," he wrote, "and stimulants and light *nourishment cautiously* administered, meet every requirement . . . . All that the dying person, then, requires is to be left alone, and allowed to die in peace."[16]

The patient's best interest is often the primary deciding factor for the physician who is considering withholding treatment.

> The withdrawing of artificial means of prolonging life . . . is not euthanasia, it is just good medicine . . . . To refrain from giving inappropriate treatment is not euthanasia either. For instance, if a man has lost a large slice of brain in a road accident, but still goes on breathing, he should not be given antibiotics to prevent infection of the wound! It is a legitimate medical judgment to decide that it is not in the interest of the patient to resuscitate him.[17]

All physicians who minister to the terminally ill are faced with an almost impossible medical ethical dilemma because they have taken an oath to relieve suffering as well as to prolong life; many times these two injunctions conflict with one another. To prolong and protect life in many instances violates the promise to relieve suffering. On the other hand, to relieve pain often violates the promise to prolong and protect the patient's life.[18] This problem presents not only an ethical dilemma, but a legal dilemma as well.

> Under present law doctors are more and more faced with the dilemma of having to choose between allowing prolonged suffering, or mercifully granting a request for death in violation of

> criminal law. This dilemma ought not to be. A reasonable and humane society should not encourage covert action by doctors in order for them to grant a terminally ill person's plea for merciful release; it should instead enact laws that would safeguard both the individual's right to live and his right to die.[19]

The Legal View

Euthanasia is illegal in the United States, Canada, and every other civilized country. Even in those countries where euthanasia is legally murder, because juries tend to sympathize with mercy killings, the law is often circumvented, making for great inequities within the legal system.[20]

> When cases of mercy killings have been brought to trial, judges and juries, moved by compassion when they learned the tragic circumstances, have almost always refused to convict the person of crime. Almost always they have found some pretext for circumventing the law, even when the evidence was clear that the person did in fact kill. Surely this is an undesirable state of affairs. If the laws are so inadequate and inhumane that compassionate people will not enforce them, it is time for new laws to be enacted . . . . What is morally right should be made legally permissible.[21]

As Richard Lamerton claims, "Legalizing euthanasia would only be acknowledging what is already going on."[22]

In 1972, Williams made a study of the 51 legal jurisdictions—50 states and the federal system—each of which has, to some extent, different rules. He was unable to find any case in which passive euthanasia was not upheld insofar as it was chosen by a competent adult. His interpretation is that the courts seem to say almost unanimously that giving medical attention to a patient who does not want it is an assault and battery and it may bring a lawsuit by the patient.[23] Morison also made a thorough search of the English-language legal literature and found not one criminal action charging that a physician omitted treatment with the intent of shortening life. Indeed, there are surprisingly few actions that charge *active* euthanasia. Even in the few cases in which charges were filed, juries have shown a reluctance to convict when there is evidence that the action was undertaken in good faith to put the patient beyond suffering.[24]

The question is sometimes raised whether there is any difference, from a legal point of view, between the actual withdrawal of treatment in progress and the withholding of treatment. Rozovsky contends that the rule in either case is that there is a duty to do what is reasonable in the circumstances. If, given the condition of the patient, it is not reasonable to resuscitate or to continue treatment, there is no duty.[25] And concerning the question of who should make this final decision for those patients incapable of making it themselves, the Massachusetts Supreme Judicial Court ruled in November of 1977 that a probate court—not a panel of doctors or other experts—should decide case-by-case whether to disconnect life-support systems from incompetent or unconscious patients.[26]

The Theological View

In the Protestant church, there are "all possible colors in the spectrum of attitudes toward euthanasia. Some condemn it, some favor it, and *many are in between, advocating judgment of each case individually.*"[27] The Catholic church condemns active euthanasia as murder and therefore a mortal sin. Lamerton, however, claims that the fact that Christian ethics are traditionally opposed to euthanasia and suicide is irrelevant, since most of our modern society is not Christian.[28] Passive medical euthanasia is treated quite differently. The church distinguishes between "ordinary" and "extraordinary" measures employed by physicians when suffering and certain death lie ahead. Pope Pius XII issued an encyclical declaring that physicians do not have to use heroic measures in such circumstances. Thus, passive euthanasia is sanctioned by the Catholic church.[29] The Orthodox Jewish view is that taking or shortening of a human life is ethically wrong, and premature termination of life or euthanasia is no less murder for the good intentions that were the motivation for the immoral act.[30]

The Hospice View

Many feel that euthanasia is preferable to dysthanasia; however, Richard Lamerton, the medical director of St. Joseph's Hospice in London, feels that the case for euthanasia is nonsense. "Because of a lack of caring in our community some people die in distress. The same lack of caring leads people to suggest euthanasia as a solution."[31] He sums up the hospice view of euthanasia in this way:

> To fail to provide for the needs of the dying is to fail in a basic duty. The self-evident requirements of a dying man are to have his symptoms relieved and to be allowed to die with dignity and peace of mind. If we evade all the difficult problems he presents,

> and just kill him, we have failed. Whether such euthanasia were voluntary or not is irrelevant. It is our duty so to care for these patients that they never ask for euthanasia. A patient who is longing to die is not being treated properly. If we are not treating him properly, the solution is to improve our treatment, not to kill him.[32]

As Cicely Saunders of St. Christopher's Hospice puts it, "The responsibility of those who oppose any form of euthanasia is to see that no one should suffer the distress that impels him to ask for it."[33] Hospice has taken on this responsibility.

In the Matter of Karen Ann Quinlan

The most dramatic right-to-die case in modern times is that of Karen Ann Quinlan. On April 15, 1975, a 21-year-old woman of Landing, New Jersey went into a coma after taking drugs and liquor. In September 1975, after they were told by doctors that there was no hope for Karen's recovery, her parents, acting with the approval of their parish priest, asked a state court for permission to authorize physicians attending their daughter to withdraw the mechanical respirator keeping her alive.[34] The court refused. Thus began a court battle unique in legal history. A father of an adult child in a persistent comatose state was seeking to be appointed guardian for the express purpose of authorizing the discontinuance of "all extraordinary procedures for sustaining his daughter's vital processes."[35]

Joseph Quinlan, a devout Catholic, appealed the decision of the Superior Court. The proceedings of the appeal to the Supreme Court of New Jersey are so thought-provoking and so closely related to the central theme of this book that the remainder of this section on euthanasia is devoted to quotations excerpted from the Decision of the Supreme Court of New Jersey In the Matter of Karen Quinlan, an Alleged Incompetent.

> The matter is of transcendent importance, involving questions related to the definition and existence of death, the prolongation of life through artificial means developed by medical technology undreamed of in past generations of the practice of the healing arts; the impact of such durationally indeterminate and artificial life prolongation on the rights of the incompetent, her family and society in general; the bearing of constitutional right and the scope of judicial responsibility, as to the appropriate response of an equity court of justice to the extraordinary prayer for relief of the plaintiff.

* * *

From all of this evidence, and including the whole testimonial record, several basic findings in the physical area are mandated. Severe brain damage and associated damage, albeit of uncertain etiology, has left Karen in a chronic and persistent vegetative state. No form of treatment which can cure or improve that condition is known or available. As nearly as may be determined, considering the guarded area of remote uncertainties characteristic of most medical science predictions, she can *never* be restored to cognitive or sapient life. Even with regard to the vegetative level of improvement therein (if such it may be called) the prognosis is extremely poor and the extent unknown if it should in fact occur.

* * *

This case is not to be considered euthanasia in any way; that would never be licit.

* * *

Competent medical testimony has established that Karen Quinlan has no reasonable hope of recovery from her comatose state by the use of any available medical procedures. The continuance of mechanical (cardiorespiratory) supportive measures to sustain continuance of her body functions and her life constitute extraordinary means of treatment. *Therefore the decision of Joseph Quinlan to request the discontinuance of this treatment is, according to the teachings of the Catholic Church, a morally correct decision.*

* * *

The claimed interests of the State in this case are essentially the preservation and sanctity of human life and defense of the right of the physician to administer medical treatment according to his best judgment. In this case the doctors say that removing Karen from the respirator will conflict with their professional judgment.

* * *

Ultimately there comes a point at which the individual's rights overcome the State interest.

* * *

We glean from the record here that physicians distinguish between curing the ill and comforting and easing the dying; that

> they refuse to treat the curable as if they were dying or ought to die, and that they have sometimes refused to treat the hopeless and dying as if they were curable . . . many of them have refused to inflict an undesired prolongation of the process of dying on a patient in irreversible condition when it is clear that such "therapy" offers neither human or humane benefit. We think these attitudes represent a balanced implementation of a profoundly realistic perspective on the meaning of life and death and that they respect the whole Judeo-Christian tradition of regard for human life.
>
> * * *
>
> The evidence in this case convinces us that the focal point of decision should be the prognosis as to the reasonable possibility of return to cognitive and sapient life, as distinguished from the forced continuance of that biological vegetative existence to which Karen seems to be doomed.
>
> * * *
>
> We do not question the State's undoubted power to punish the taking of human life, but that power does not encompass individuals terminating medical treatment pursuant to their right of privacy.[36]

Thus, on March 31, 1976, almost a year after Karen had entered her comatose state, the Supreme Court of New Jersey ruled that Joseph Quinlan was the guardian of her person, and thus she was removed from the mechanical life support systems. Miraculously, she has been able to breathe on her own, and at this writing, more than two years later, although she has never gained consciousness, she is a living and breathing human being in a vegetative state.

SUICIDE

Every day in the United States, about 60 people kill themselves by poisoning, hanging, drowning, shooting, stabbing, jumping from high places, or other means.[37] About 25,000 suicides are reported each year, but the actual number is much higher, probably twice the reported rate. Suicide attempts are about eight times the number of reported suicides.[38] Worldwide, more than 500,000 suicides are registered yearly, according to the World Health Organization, and there are approximately eight times as many suicide attempts.[39]

> Several salient features of the problem deserve mention. Suicides are three times as frequent in men than in women although there are more attempts by women than men. Twice as many White Americans commit suicide than do Negro Americans and twice as many single people kill themselves than do married individuals. College students have a suicide rate 50% higher than non-college students of comparable age, sex and race. In industrialized countries physicians, dentists and lawyers have a higher rate of suicide than other professionals. Although the suicide rate has remained relatively constant in the United States over the past decade or so, poisoning by drugs, especially barbiturates, has become much more popular as a method of choice. The age group with the highest suicide rate is that above 65 years. Suicide ranks third as a cause of death among teenagers. It has also been estimated that the ratio of suicide attempts to actual successes in adolescents is one hundred to one.[40]

Generally, under Orthodox Jewish law, a suicide is not accorded full burial honors. Rending one's garments, delivering memorial addresses and other rites of mourning that are an honor for the dead are not to be performed for a suicide victim.[41] Islamic law forbids suicide. The act is viewed by Islam as a form of murder, and, therefore, since murder is evil, suicide must also be forbidden. Islamics feel that paradise will be denied the offender. Catholics who commit suicide are often afforded funeral rites on the assumption that the victims were not in possession of their faculties at the time, hence not responsible for the act.[42]

Assisting a suicide is illegal in every country except Uruguay.[43] Although suicide is not legally a crime in most American jurisdictions, aiding and abetting suicide is murder. In England, the 1961 Suicide Act states that it is not a criminal offense for people, whether in sickness or in health, to take their own lives or to attempt to do so. However, any individual who helps a person commit suicide is liable to a charge of manslaughter.[44]

Joseph Fletcher, in his provocative treatise *Morals and Medicine* proclaimed:

> Sometimes patients *in extremis* try to outwit the doctors and escape from medicine's ministrations. They swallow Kleenex to suffocate themselves, or jerk tubes out of their noses or veins, in a cat-and-mouse game of life and death which is neither merciful nor meaningful. Medical innovation makes it ever easier to drag people back to life in merely physiological terms. Yet when these

> patients succeed in outwitting their medical ministrants, can we say that they have committed suicide in any real sense of the word? Who is actually alive in these contrivances and contraptions? In such a puppetlike state most patients are, of course, too weakened and drugged to take any truly human initiative.[45]

NO-CODE ORDERS

Suddenly the hospital's paging system blares, "Code blue to ICU!" This cryptic message is repeated three times, and before the echoes in the corridors die out, a team of specially trained experts have rushed to the intensive care unit (ICU), where a patient has undergone a cardiac arrest. Depending upon the specific institution, the paging code might have been "Dr. Heart," "Dr. Heartstone," "Blue Code," or some other generic signal that generates the same immediate response.

The team generally consists of nurses, inhalation therapists, pulmonary technician, cardiologist, pulmonary physiologist, possibly an anesthesiologist, and others, whose prime function is to provide the patient with cardiopulmonary resuscitation (CPR).

> The purpose of CPR is the prevention of sudden unexpected death. CPR is not indicated in certain situations, such as in cases of terminal irreversible illness where death is not unexpected or where prolonged cardiac arrest dictates the futility of resuscitative efforts. Resuscitation in these circumstances may represent a positive violation of an individual's right to die with dignity.[46]

Probably the only therapeutic modality that can be initiated in a health care facility without a physician's order is CPR, when cardiac or respiratory arrest is recognized. A specific instruction by the patient's physician is necessary if CPR is *not* to be initiated. This instruction in the patient's chart is usually indicated by "no code," "do not code," "no code blue," "do not resuscitate," or similar wording. " 'Code blue' may be defined as those acute measures which rescue the patient from momentarily impending and otherwise inevitable death."[47]

According to Garth Tagge, therapy orders in the ICU are often unrealistic and frequently prolong the process of dying or are insufficient for survival. "Half treatment of a critically ill patient is illogical and must be avoided."[48] He says that these unrealistic orders are of three types: 1) do everything you can, but if patient arrests, do not resuscitate; 2) if the patient bleeds, give a transfusion; 3) give antibiotics and steroids but not parenteral nutrition.[49] Thus, the main question is, when is a patient actually terminal? The no-code decision must be preceded by the conclusion that the patient is suffering a terminal condition. When time permits, this may be a joint decision made by the patient, family, friends, clergy, and all of the members of the medical care team, but the final decision must be left to the coordinator of the patient's care—the physician.[50]

After code blue is instituted, there is still another decision to be made—that is, when reasonable resuscitation efforts have failed. Again, all the medical factors must be taken into consideration, and the final decision to cease resuscitation efforts must be made by the best qualified individual—the coordinator of the medical team, the physician, or in the physician's absence, the resuscitation team leader.[51] Rozovsky feels that every health care facility should have a standing rule that a no-code order be reviewed on a periodic short time basis and that any change in the patient's condition upon which the order might have been based be immediately reported to the physician so that the opinion might be reassessed.[52]

Patients, if they wish, have a legal right to refuse treatment so that they may die naturally. There have been no reported court decisions holding a physician liable for failure to resuscitate a terminally ill patient. When the conscious patient and the family are in agreement, the legal risk seems minimal.[53]

Many feel that nurses should not be expected to act on oral no-code orders. By contrast, George Annas tells us that at Massachusetts General Hospital the policy is that DNR (do not resuscitate) orders are given orally to nursing and house staff and noted in nursing notes, but not written into the regular order sheet or permanent record. He contends that until 1975, when the law was changed, nursing notes were routinely destroyed following the patient's death or discharge. The only purpose of such a policy was to destroy any evidence that the physician ever gave such an order or that the hospital approved the order.[54] Such a procedure can only intensify public distrust of the medical profession.

Until recent years there was great hugger-mugger in hospital circles about no-code orders. The issue becomes quite emotional when, upon occasion, the press reports that a patient died and that a no-code order had been written in the patient's chart. A Canadian newspaper reported that the Canadian Medical Association atttracted much attention when it adopted the position that it is ethical for physicians to write "no resuscitation" on a patient's chart when they believe that the patient is facing "impending, inevitable death."[55]

Probably the most spectacular brouhaha surrounding this topic began with the Los Angeles County coroner's inquest held on the body of Raymond S. Oden, August 30 and 31, 1977. Oden, aged 64, had been a ward of the Los Angeles County Public Guardian's Office. He had been a patient in the Community Care Center, a convalescent facility located in Duarte, California, Los Angeles County, when, on July 28, 1977, he became quite nauseous and began vomiting. He was transferred on July 29, 1977 to the Monrovia Community Hospital ICU where he died within hours. During the course of the inquest, which was conducted by Frederick S. Lacey, chief of the coroner's inquest division, the term *no-code* was introduced from the patient's medical record.

This came to the attention of Supervisor Baxter Ward, one of the five men making up the board of supervisors that governs mammoth Los Angeles County's 7,000,000 citizens. On September 21, 1977, Ward called a special hearing on no-code orders. During the hearing, Lacey testified that in the course of conducting over 600 inquests he had never come across the term *no-code*. When asked by Supervisor Ward how he felt the hospital staff had interpreted the no-code order, Lacey responded:

> Mr. Supervisor, this was one of the big issues as far as I was concerned. I really wasn't satisfied that [everyone] interpreted the "no-code" order in the same manner. What I'm trying to say is that there wasn't any set pattern as to its interpretation by anyone. I heard some of them testify, for example, that it meant one thing, that if they were asked, I believe, by the District Attorney, "if you had a 'no-code' order, would that mean that you would stop all treatment, for example, such as any of the medication that the doctor prescribed?" Some of them said "no." Most of them agreed it meant no heroic measures, but I was not satisfied that anyone had any absolute definite definition of what it meant.[56]

Expert medical testimony at the hearing determined that the no-code order written on patient Oden was inappropriate and that it might have prevented certain procedures from being taken to help the patient.

Ward, after hearing from at least 15 witnesses, concluded that some safeguards are needed to prevent the possibility of this kind of situation developing again in Los Angeles County or in the state of California. Therefore, on September 27, 1977 a select citizens committee was established by the board of supervisors to determine community practice regarding no-code orders and to determine if standards covering this type of action should be promulgated. At this writing, the committee is still debating the issues.

Incidentally, the verdict of the jury at the coroner's inquest into Oden's death was, death at the hands of another other than by accident.[57] On March 30, 1978 John S. Corbin was charged with involuntary manslaughter in the death of Raymond Oden.[58]

SUMMARY

An individual's right to die is as sacred as the right to live. How and when that death takes place is of great concern not only to the dying person and the family, but also to physicians, attorneys, theologians, and academicians—in short, to society. Questions are raised when death is possibly hastened by the withholding of some action that might forestall the actual moment of death (passive euthanasia), or by an action that will induce death for the purpose of terminating suffering or a meaningless existence (active euthanasia). And yet, because euthanasia is illegal and is considered by many people to be immoral, some terminally ill patients turn to their only option to achieve a peaceful death—suicide.

If more terminally ill patients and their families knew about the concepts of hospice as a caring community, there would be less concern about euthanasia and suicide. The compassionate caring and elimination of pain and suffering makes hospice the logical choice for care of the terminally ill patient.

NOTES

1. O. Ruth Russell, *Freedom To Die* (New York: Human Sciences Press, 1975), p. 232.
2. Roland Stevens, "Euthanasia: A Doctor Speaks . . . ," Address delivered at organizing meeting of the Euthanasia Educational Fund, Rochester, New York chapter, February 4, 1971.
3. Frank Veith et al., "Brain Death: I. A Status Report of Medical and Ethical Considerations," *JAMA* 238 (October 10, 1977): 1,651–5.
4. *Legislative Newsletter* (New York: Society for the Right to Die), Summer 1977, p. 2.
5. C. S. Mihanovich, "Euthanasia," *World Book Encyclopedia,* 1967.
6. Russell, p. 22.
7. Ibid.
8. Joseph Fletcher, in *Death and Decisions: Excerpts from Papers and Discussion at the 7th Annual Euthanasia Conference* (New York: The Euthanasia Educational Council, December 7, 1974), p. 7.
9. Ibid.

10. Glanville Williams, "Euthanasia Legislation: A Rejoinder to the Non-Religious Objections," in *Euthanasia and the Right to Die,* ed. A. B. Downing (London: Peter Owen, 1969), pp. 134–47.

11. Emil Freireich, in *Death and Decisions,* p. 20.

12. Mary Rose Barrington, "Apologia for Suicide," in *Euthanasia and the Right to Die,* pp. 152–72.

13. Ibid.

14. A. B. Downing, "Euthanasia: The Human Context," in *Euthanasia and the Right to Die,* pp. 13–24.

15. *AMA Council Guidelines for Physicians on Euthanasia* (Chicago: American Medical Association, 1973).

16. William Munk, *Euthanasia: or Medical Treatment in Aid of an Easy Death* (London: Longmans, Green & Co., 1887), pp. 86–7.

17. Lamerton, *Care of the Dying* (Westport, Connecticut: Technomic Publishing Co., 1976), pp. 89–90.

18. Joseph Fletcher, *Morals and Medicine* (Boston: Beacon, 1960), p. 172.

19. Russell, p. 10.

20. Rosner, p. 110.

21. Russell, pp. 218 and 235.

22. Lamerton, p. 89.

23. C. Dickerman Williams, in *Death and Decisions*, p. 25.

24. Robert A. Morison, "Dying," *Life and Death and Medicine: A Scientific American Book* (San Francisco: Freeman, 1973), pp. 39–45.

25. Lorne E. Rozovsky, "Resuscitation and the Euthanasia Debate," *Dimensions in Health Service* 52 (November 1975): 8–9.

26. Patrick R. Carroll, "Who Speaks for Incompetent Patients? The Case of Joseph Saikewicz," *Trustee* 31 (December 1978): 19–24.

27. Fred Rosner, *Studies in Torah Judaism: Modern Medicine and Jewish Law* (New York: Yeshiva University, 1972), p. 115.

28. Lamerton, p. 92.

29. Rosner, pp. 114–5.

30. Veith et al., loc. cit.

31. Lamerton, p. 100.

32. Lamerton, p. 95.

33. Cicely Saunders, "Care for the Dying," *Patient Care* 3 (June 1976).

34. James Goodman, "New Jersey, Death and the Law," *1976 Yearbook Covering the Year 1975* (New York: Collier, 1975), p. 374.

35. Supreme Court of New Jersey, Decision in the Matter of Karen Quinlan, an Alleged Incompetent, Argued January 26, 1976, Decided March 31, 1976.

36. Ibid.

37. Rosner, p. 178.

38. Edwin Shneidman, *Deaths of Man* (Baltimore: Penguin Books, 1974), p. 33.

39. Rosner, loc. cit.

40. Rosner, pp. 178–9.

41. Ibid., p. 193.
42. Corinne L. Hatton, Sharon M. Valente, and Alice Rink, eds., *Suicide: Assessment and Intervention* (New York: Appleton-Century-Crofts, 1977), p. 7.
43. Lamerton, p. 90.
44. Rosner, p. 109.
45. Fletcher, *Morals and Medicine,* p. 65.
46. "Standards for Cardiopulmonary Resuscitation and Emergency Cardiac Care," *JAMA* 227 (Supplement) (February 18, 1974): 833–68.
47. "'Code' or 'No Code'", *The Bulletin,* Los Angeles County Medical Association, February 16, 1978, p. 16.
48. Garth Tagge, "Critical Care: A Classification System for ICU Patients," *The Hospital Medical Staff* 5 (February 1976): 1–6.
49. Ibid.
50. "'Code' or 'No Code'", loc. cit.
51. Ibid.
52. Rozovsky, loc. cit.
53. Richard P. Bergen, "Management of Terminal Illness," *JAMA* 229 (September 2, 1978): 1,352–3.
54. George J. Annas, "The Legal Aspects of a Patient Care Classification System," *The Hospital Medical Staff* 5 (February 1976): 12–18.
55. *Toronto Globe and Mail,* June 24, 1975.
56. Testimony of Frederick S. Lacey at special Los Angeles County Board of Supervisors hearing on no-code orders, September 21, 1977.
57. Ibid.
58. "Doctor Charged in Man's Death," *Los Angeles Times,* March 31, 1978, part II, p. 5.

Chapter 6

Hospice: A Caring Community

To live without feeling or exciting sympathy, to be fortunate without adding to the felicity of others, or afflicted without tasting the balm of pity, is a state more gloomy than solitude: it is not retreat, but exclusion from mankind.
Samuel Johnson, *Rasselas*

Attend a workshop or meeting with hospice-interested people, and a sense of camaraderie pervades the setting. Not only are old friendships renewed, but the feeling of sharing, and an indescribable sensitivity brought about by dealing with death, ripple through the discussions both at the formal sessions and at the informal social gatherings. This sense of sharing is different and more intense than I have found at similar gatherings of hospital-interested people. There is also no comparable tone in meetings of those who do not provide personal services in their everyday lives. Barbara Hill, former executive director of Hospice of Marin, described this special hospice feeling beautifully at the Third National Hospice Symposium:

> My belief is that a specific environment needs to be created to develop a hospice—that of the love relationship. I believe that in a truly accepting, undemanding love environment the source exists for growth of the individual. It matters not whether that love is the love of husband and wife, therapist and client, mother and child, or hospice staff member and hospice family—when that mutual love and trust develop, miracles happen.[1*]

Plant contends that "hospices are gaining favor in the U.S. because they are a curious amalgam of reactions and responses." She claims that one reaction is against the cure-at-any-cost syndrome that pervades the acute-care hospital. Another is the rebellion against hospital regulations that tend to keep patients and families apart in times of crisis. A third reaction is against certain of society's attitudes about death that prevent

*Reprinted by permission from "Alternative Models of Hospice Care," Barbara Hill, by permission of Hospice of Marin, Marin Co., California.

the provision of the best care to the dying. The responses are all part of the slowly emerging movement toward death with dignity and the search for alternatives to institutionalization.[2]

All programs that care for the dying and their families are not necessarily hospice programs.[3] "A hospice is not a hospital and not a nursing home. The hospice is inspired by a different philosophy of care, relates to different goals, and provides different services to an entirely different population of cancer patients."[4] The hospice concept does not suggest a deficit in hospital care, but rather recognizes the fact that neither general, teaching, nor research hospitals are staffed for and oriented to providing care for terminally ill patients.[5]

HOSPICE MODELS

As noted earlier, a hospice is not necessarily an institution; a hospice is a program of care. It may be a home care program, a free-standing institution, a separate hospital department, or an interdisciplinary team that moves within a general hospital to wherever the patients may be located within the facility. It may offer outpatient services or day care; it may offer the home care in conjunction with the institutional settings, or it might combine variations of these models. A controversy is currently brewing over which of these models is the best for terminally ill patients. There is, however, no one "best" model.

Home Care and Institutional Hospice Services

Most people, given the choice, would prefer to die at home. Hence, home care hospice services seem to be most appropriate. Yet, a point may come in the home care regimen when the patient may have to be sent to an institutional hospice for a time to control new symptoms, provide the psychological boost of a fresh environment, or to provide relief and rest for the family members who must provide 24-hour-per-day aid to the patient.

The patient, then, will be transferred to the institutional hospice for a few days before being returned to the home and familiar surroundings so important to the terminally ill.

> The dying have the right to a great many things that hospitals and nursing homes simply cannot provide. They need life around them, spiritual and emotional comfort and support of every sort. They need "unsanitary" things, like a favorite dog lying at the foot of the bed. They need their own clothes, their own pictures, music, food, surroundings that are familiar to them, people they

know and love, people they can trust to care about them. Hospices can provide this in their inpatient units; and yet, for many individuals and their families, it is much better for it to happen at home.[6]

Free-Standing Versus Hospital-Based Hospices

At this writing, the National Cancer Institute has provided funding for three separate free-standing hospices. At this writing, only one is operative: Hillhaven Hospice in Tucson, Arizona. Under construction is Hospice, Inc. in New Haven, Connecticut, and to become operational by mid-to-late 1978 is Kaiser-Permanente Medical Care Program in Los Angeles. Although British hospices are almost exclusively free-standing, it appears unlikely that United States hospices will emerge as free-standing facilities.

Several additional free-standing facilities will probably be built in the future, but growth of the movement will depend on expansion of the home care- and the hospital-based models. Home care-based hospices will grow because of the inherent cost-saving features, and hospital-based hospices will proliferate because of the excess hospital beds available throughout the country. Because of the excess hospital beds, capital construction funds are and will be extremely difficult to obtain. Lawrence Burke of the National Cancer Institute feels that "it would more than compromise and complicate the [hospice] program to have it initiated within a general hospital."[7] On the other hand, Balfour Mount of the Royal Victoria Hospital questions the economic feasibility of free-standing hospices. "Analysis of the economics of maintaining such institutions . . . suggests that society cannot afford to support an adequate number to meet the need."[8]

A major objection to the hospital-based hospice unit is the almost diametrically opposed philosophies of *acute* care and *palliative* care. Opponents reason that the terminally ill patients are torn apart by observing hospital patients who will be leaving the hospital in the matter of a few days well on the road to recovery. To be in a hospital and know that patients in other parts of the hospital will be *cured* of their illnesses is a tremendous psychological barrier to the effective care of the hospice patients. Then, too, the acute-care training of personnel has run counter to that needed for hospice care. Hospital personnel will frequently refer to the hospice unit as the "dead end," or they may make other disparaging remarks that only serve to antagonize the hospice personnel and that may result in counter productivity to the type of care to be provided to hospice patients.

The Mixed-Community Hospice

A 1950 study of cancer patients concluded that facilities for the care of terminal cancer patients should not be set up as specialized institutions operated solely for the care of *cancer* patients, as places where patients go to die from cancer. The report wisely proclaimed that, "specialization of this type is almost inhuman in the emotional trauma it produces for the patient and his family."[9] British hospices do not care only for the terminally ill, nor do they concentrate only on problems associated with advanced cancer. For example, St. Joseph's Hospice in Hackney, London has always had a well-mixed community of patients, and it has a home care program in its geographical area for anyone dying of anything. It also has a unit for long-term rehabilitation and home support. St. Christopher's Hospice in Sydenham, London has a wing for frail elderly and has a number of longer-stay patients with various diagnoses in its wards.[10]

APPROPRIATE TREATMENT

The distinction between appropriate and inappropriate treatment of patients is a paramount concern of hospices. "This distinction means concentration on control of symptoms when definitive treatment for disease is no longer possible," writes Sylvia Lack. She adds that the best way to do this is with a centrally coordinated service of in-patient beds and a home care program under an autonomous hospice administration.[11] When a person's life is in its last few hours, that person needs a quiet place in which to die naturally. Most patients in a hospice die peacefully with no intravenous injections or gastric tubes, but if such treatment is appropriate, it is used.[12]

Patients come to hospices only when they have terminal illnesses that can no longer be treated or cured. The omission of further surgery or radiotherapy for these patients is the omission of extraordinary and optional means of prolonging the dying process. Thus, hospices do not practice dysthanasia; they practice JUCTO (justifiable use of conservative therapy only).[13]

> Formerly, when most people died at home, children grew up with a realistic understanding of death from which they are now shielded. Yet watching someone die in the loving and caring surrounding of a hospice surely does less emotional damage to a young child than watching even one evening of television violence.[14]

Britain's 30-odd hospices are homelike places of care where terminally ill patients, with or without money, are given everything possible to allow them to die with dignity and to avoid unnecessary prolongation of life. The hospices are constantly developing new techniques to reduce pain, and doctors and nurses are devoting their entire careers to furthering this aim.[15]

ELEMENTS OF A HOSPICE PROGRAM

The most common indication for admission to hospices—in some 40 percent of cases—is the need to give respite to relatives. On the other hand, 20 percent of admissions are social isolates with no one able or willing to care for them. At the same time, 60 percent of admissions need help with better control of their pain. Thus, hospice patients represent a mix of social and clinical need.[16]

A hospice program, then, is not just a program that purports to care for the terminally ill. It is a program for meeting a wide range of physical, psychological, social, and spiritual needs, a program of health care delivery consisting of ten clearly identifiable elements:

1. Service availability to home care patients and inpatients on a 24-hour-a-day, seven-day-a-week, on-call basis with emphasis on availability of medical and nursing skills
2. Home care service in collaboration with inpatient facilities
3. Knowledge and expertise in the control of symptoms (physical, psychological, social, and spiritual)
4. The provision of care by an interdisciplinary team
5. Physician-directed services
6. Central administration and coordination of services
7. Use of volunteers as an integral part of the health care team
8. Acceptance to the program based on health needs, not ability to pay
9. Treatment of the patient and family together as the unit of care
10. A bereavement follow-up service[17]

Not all existing hospice programs incorporate all ten of these elements. For example, some are entirely home care oriented, while others are exclusively institution based with no home care services; some have very limited bereavement follow-up service, while others have extensive bereavement service; many have services available on a 24-hour-a-day, seven-day-a-week basis, while some have more limited hours. Nevertheless, the ten elements represent the ideal to be achieved by any hospice program.

Home Care Plus Inpatient Services

The goal of hospice care is to help a patient continue life as usual—working, being with a family, doing what is especially significant before life comes to a close, and feeling a part of the ongoing life—not being different. Much of this type of care is fostered through the home care and outpatient programs. Hospices place primary emphasis on home care so that patients can maintain their life styles as long as possible, but they usually supplement the home care with their own inpatient unit, or they may have an arrangement with a local palliative-care hospital unit. The practical needs are to relieve families for a while, to provide 24-hour medical supervision when symptoms cannot be controlled at home, and to guarantee the professional care that is necessary during the final weeks of life. The overriding ideological and practical need, however, is continuity of care, for without a hospice-run inpatient unit, patients must enter hospitals or nursing homes and lose touch with the special symptom-control measures and medication regimens that typify hospice care.[18] The knowledge that a hospice bed is available in the inpatient facility often makes it possible for the patient to remain at home longer than either the family or the patient consider possible.

Emotional and Psychological Support

Emotional and psychological support is as essential an element of care as symptom control. Each patient is seen as part of a family unit, whose total well-being and lifestyle affect and are affected by care. Flexibility geared to the patient's mental and physical comfort characterizes the inpatient unit. Visiting hours are flexible (usually 24 hours per day), very young children and even pets are welcome at any time, meals are provided on demand, and wine and liquor are served in moderation. Patients also wear their own clothing and can bring favorite possessions, including furniture from home.[19]

In an article in the popular press, English hospice residents were described as being able to move about and enjoy days filled with a variety of activities, including art classes, pottery, crafts, bingo games, musical entertainment by volunteers, gardening, and automobile drives. All this while the patients were heavily dosed with pain-killing narcotics—yet most seemed alert.[20] For the patient with too much time to think, the systematic use of games of all kinds, under the supervision of the occupational therapist, is necessary.

In English hospices, even mealtime is a social event. Sherry or beer is always served before the meals. This stimulates the appetite and relaxes the patient as well as contributes to the nutritional state. Each course is then brought in separately and served to the patient in small portions. The nurse or volunteer takes the necessary care and time to make the patient feel wanted. This is unlike American hospitals, where large portions of food are placed on a tray in front of the patient, and personnel return in one-half to three-fourths of an hour to remove the usually uneaten meal.[21]

In an age of specialization and fragmentation, when a variety of medical specialists may be fascinated by the disease process and forget the patient, it falls to the nurse to reaffirm the personal identity and unique worth of the patient. However, care must be exercised that the staff address the patients as adults who understand. It is all too easy to talk down to patients, as though they were children or mentally deficient.[22] If this is done, the patient's emotional needs will not be met and all the good work of the hospice will be undone.

Little things are important, such things as washing a patient's hair, helping the patient to write a letter, moving the bed closer to the window to afford a better view of outdoor activities; these services can all be performed by either nursing personnel or volunteers. And of course physical touch is extremely important. Holding hands, caressing the face, stroking the hair—these are all forms of intimate communication, communication that does not depend on the spoken word. These continual personal reassurances to the dying patient speak of love, deep compassionate love between human beings.

The Interdisciplinary Team Approach

Fundamental to the hospice concept is the interdisciplinary team approach. No one person has all the answers to the problems of the dying patient and the family; such problems are multitudinous. The team is usually headed by a clinical physician. "The hospice program of care usually is directed by a physician for two reasons: first, symptom control, the focus of hospice care, is a medical concern, and second, a medical director is best able to generate understanding and support for the hospice concept among other physicians."[23]

It is the physician who gives general direction to members of the other disciplines—nurses, social workers, chaplains, physiotherapists, psychiatrists, dieticians, pharmacists, and volunteers. The composition of the interdisciplinary team will, of course, differ with each hospice.

> Clearly the roles of doctor, priest and nurse are not going to be in neat compartments, for at times they will be completely interchangeable. To be instantly responsive to the patient's needs, one requires nurses who can alter the dosage of drugs, recognize when to give a wide range of "when necessary" prescriptions, and insert a urinary catheter. One needs doctors who can also be spiritual advisers and clergymen who can competently impart a grave prognosis. It is the widening of the scope of one's work, closer to the traditional role of the old-time family doctor, which is the principal attraction in care of the dying.[24]

Because the physician, the psychiatrist, and the nurse have acquired the image of being too busy, the person whom the patient and family frequently confide in about their deepest concerns is the volunteer, who is seen as the one person who has time and understanding.[25] Volunteers are utilized both in inpatient and home care programs. There are no standards for numbers of volunteers who might be used in various programs, but for home care programs a ratio of 12 lay volunteers to each professional is suggested.[26]

The legal counselor can be an important part of the interdisciplinary team. An attorney can help with legal, financial, or estate-planning needs, drafting the documents necessary to guarantee that patients' dependents will be sensibly provided for. Patients will then at least have peace of mind knowing that their wishes will be honored and that their loved ones will be protected.[27]

When unpleasant symptoms are under control and the patient is able to return home from the hospice facility for a time, then a social worker can be the liaison between the two and can help to deal with the economic consequences of a disease that has destroyed a person's earning capacity. All financial worries should be resolved before the death.[28]

Some of the team members may experience the "burn-out" phenomenon, especially the nursing personnel. Dealing with death, becoming intensely involved emotionally with patients and their families day after day, can affect a care giver psychologically and emotionally. The emotional drain caused by several deaths occurring in a relatively short period of time can take its toll in pent-up emotions screaming to be released; therefore, some hospice facilities are providing "scream rooms" to provide this release. Jerry Coash, director of the Encino Hospital palliative care unit, explained that he copes with this problem by having the nurses who spend the majority of their time in the hospice unit occasionally rotated to other nursing units within the hospital, even though continuity suffers.[29]

The Family as Patient

To the hospice team, the "patient" is undeniably the patient and the family. The family, in the broad sense, includes not only the natural family (immediate and other relatives), but also the extended family (natural family plus friends, and even pets) and the adopted family (the care givers).[30] Figure 6-1 shows the relationship of the elements of care to the unit of care: the terminally ill patient and the family.

Naturally, some relatives will be part of the caring team, some will be patients along with the dying person, while others will alternate between the two roles. It may be that they will need to be put up in the facility overnight, if they are too distressed to return home alone, or if they want to be close at hand when death is imminent.[31]

Because they are also patients, relatives need to be cared for as well. For this reason, some hospices have a "relative's day off," when visiting of all but the most severely ill patients is discouraged. This releases the friend or relative who feels a duty to be visiting the loved one as much as possible and who consequently never gets out. Otherwise, visiting is unrestricted.[32]

The death of a person should leave the family with no feelings that they did not do enough. They should be directly involved in the patient's care. The team can teach the family various health care measures that will enable the patient to remain at home and, when inpatient care becomes necessary, should encourage the family to participate in that care too, by helping the nurses with feeding, turning, washing, and so on. Since this is their last offering, they want to be as close as possible to their loved one.[33]

Bereavement Services

Since grief begins at the moment when the patient's illness is diagnosed as terminal, relatives should not be told of this condition and then left to their own devices. They should be invited to come back and talk over their distress and to ask questions.[34] "To support a family through grieving before and after bereavement demands understanding and tolerance from the care givers. Understanding implies a familiarity with the patterns

Figure 6-1 The Hospice in Patient Care

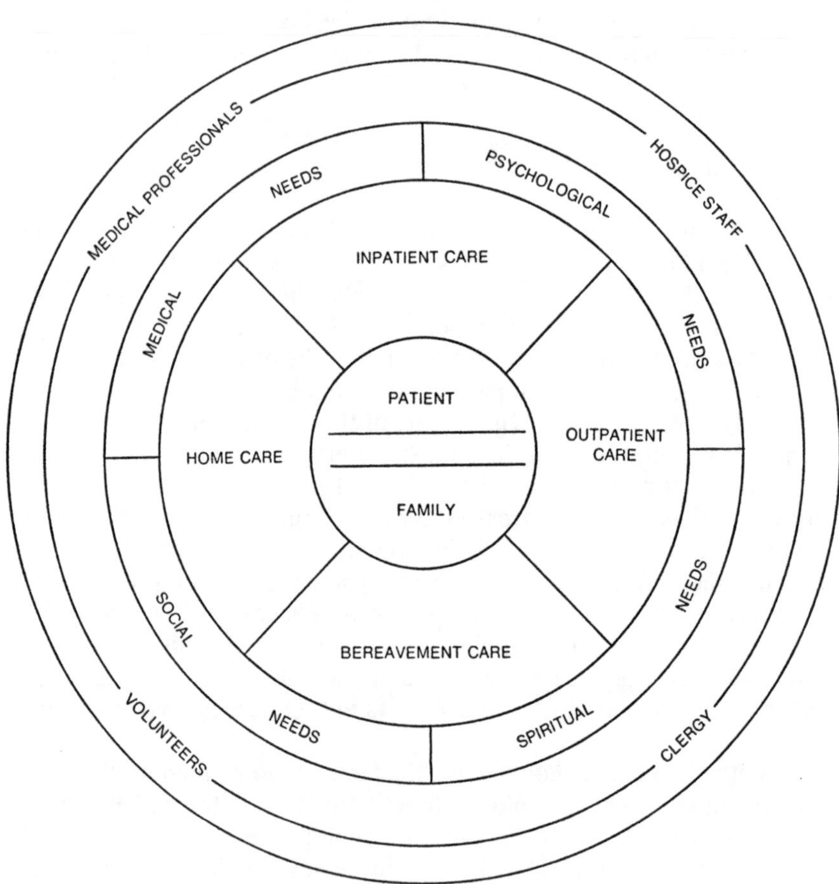

Source: "The Hospice Movement," Management Services Special Report, unpublished (Newport Beach, California: Advanced Health Systems, Inc., October 1977), p. 4. Reprinted by permission of Advanced Health Systems, Inc., 881 Dover Drive, Suite 20, Newport Beach, California 92663.

---

and processes of normal grief, while tolerance implies a capacity to accept the variable forms the process may assume."[35]

Bereavement follow-up is an essential part of hospice care. Follow-up can last for any length of time and take various forms, including home visits by team members who had treated the patient, phone calls, notes, or assisting a lonely spouse in finding a job. Such follow-up helps to support not only the family at a time when its members are particularly vulnerable to physical and psychological stress, but also the hospice team, which has also suffered a loss in the death of a patient.[36] William Lamers, in an interview describing the operation of Hospice of Marin, stated, "When our nurses and counselors have worked with a family and ultimately death occurs, each individual who worked with that family attends the funeral. Then we see that families are followed by our nurses and counselors for a period of at least a year after death has occurred."[37]

In a hospice there are often a number of bereaved people who are working through their grief by doing voluntary work for a few months following the death.[38] Thus, this activity is therapeutic for the survivors. Yet most hospices permit this only for a period of, say, six months to a year after death.

NOTES

1. Barbara Hill, "The 'How To' of Hospice Care," Proceedings of the Third National Hospice Symposium, Dominican College Campus, San Rafael, California, May 26–28, 1977, p. 18.
2. Janet Plant, "Finding a Home for Hospice Care in the U.S.," *Hospitals, JAHA* 51 (July 1, 1977): 53–62.
3. Sylvia Lack, "I Want To Die While I'm Still Alive," *Death Education* 1, no. 2 (Summer 1977): 165–76.
4. Letter from Lawrence D. Burke, Program Director for Rehabilitation Treatment, Rehabilitation and Continuing Care Branch (DCCR), National Cancer Institute, HEW, December 15, 1977.
5. Ibid.
6. Sandol Stoddard citing William Lamers, *The Hospice Movement: A Better Way of Caring for the Dying* (Briarcliff Manor, N.Y.: Stein and Day, 1978), p. 51.
7. Burke letter.
8. Balfour M. Mount, "The Problem of Caring for the Dying in a General Hospital: The Palliative Care Unit As a Possible Solution," *Canadian Medical Association Journal* 115 (July 17, 1976): 119–21.
9. *Terminal Care for Cancer Patients* (Chicago: Central Service for the Chronically Ill of the Institute of Medicine of Chicago, 1950), p. 15.
10. St. Christopher's Hospice, "Annual Report, 1976–1977," p. 12.
11. Lack, loc. cit.
12. Ibid.
13. D. G. McCarthy, "Should Catholic Hospitals Sponsor Hospices?" *Hospital Progress* 57 (December 1976): 61–5.
14. Ibid.
15. Richard Kolbe, "Inside the English Hospice," *Hospitals* 51 (July 1, 1977): 65–7.
16. E. Wilkes, "Terminal Care and the Special Nursing Unit," *Nursing Times* 71 (January 9, 1975): 57–9.

17. Sylvia Lack, "Philosophy and Organization of a Hospice Program," Unpublished paper, n.d.; "I Want To Die," loc. cit.

18. Plant, loc. cit.

19. Ibid.

20. Michael Satchell, "How to Enjoy Life—Up to the Last Moment," *Parade*, October 16, 1977.

21. M. A. Rose and Walter J. Pories, "Some Additional Notes on Hospice," *Ohio State Medical Journal* 73 (June 1977), 379–82.

22. *Palliative Care Service: October 1976 Report* (Montreal: Royal Victoria Hospital, McGill University, 1976), p. 75.

23. Plant, loc. cit.

24. Richard Lamerton, *Care of the Dying* (Westport, Connecticut: Technomic Publishing Co., 1976), p. 22.

25. Lack, "I Want to Die," loc. cit.

26. Burke letter.

27. Barton E. Bernstein, "Lawyer and Counselor As an Interdisciplinary Team: Interfacing for the Terminally Ill," *Death Education* 1 (Fall 1977): 277–91.

28. Lamerton, p. 21.

29. "Hospice Care—A New Concept for the Care of the Terminally Ill and Their Families," Workshop at UCLA Extension, Los Angeles, April 8–9, 1978.

30. Robert Woodson, "The Concept of Hospice Care in Terminal Disease," *Breast Cancer*, ed. J. M. Vaeth (Basel, Switzerland: Karger, 1976), pp. 161–79.

31. Lamerton, p. 20.

32. Ibid., p. 21.

33. Ibid., p. 40

34. Lamerton, p. 125.

35. *Palliative Care Service*, p. 84.

36. Plant, loc. cit.

37. "Hospice," Interview with William Lamers, Jr., Medical Director, Hospice of Marin, *Thanatos*, March 1977, pp. 6–11.

38. Lamerton, p. 129.

Chapter 7
Contemporary Facilities for the Terminally Ill

Extreme remedies are very appropriate for extreme diseases.
Hippocrates, *Aphorisms*

Inpatient hospices are alternatives to the facilities presently accommodating terminally ill patients, i.e., hospitals and nursing homes. Although at first glance all three kinds of facilities may appear to be similar, there are stark differences, due primarily to variations in attitude and philosophy rather than to architectural and cosmetic variations.

HOSPITALS

Sir Thomas Browne wrote in *Religio Medici* II, "for the world, I count it not an inn, but an hospital, and a place, not to live, but to die in." Thus was the view of hospitals in the mid 1600s—a place in which to die. To be admitted to a hospital was to admit that death was close at hand. Florence Nightingale wrote in 1863 that the very first requirement of a hospital is that it should do the sick no harm.[1] Today, by contrast, most hospitals are places of efficiency in disease control and are furnished and designed for rapid patient turnover and efficient medical and nursing staff performance.[2] Modern general hospitals are committed not to death, but to restoring health and life.[3]

Most hospitals are social institutions constructed to provide acute remedial care. Then to ask the same social institution to provide chronic supportive care is to place the hospital staff in a double bind. To which priorities do they respond? Hospital staff do not necessarily ignore dying patients, but they give priority to patients for whom they can provide life-saving measures. This is not unreasonable, considering their training and the emphasis on curative functions rather than the caring functions needed by the dying.[4]

Here we have a dilemma in that acute-care hospitals are not well equipped to care for the dying, and as a result the dying are isolated, ignored, and left with little human contact.[5] They are perhaps given good technical care, but their actual needs many times are not recognized.

The Hospital Atmosphere

The big general hospital is not a very good place to die. Even though such hospitals have large staffs, most of these professionals are preoccupied with administrative matters and with the increasingly complicated technical aspects of keeping patients alive. Surrounded by these busy bodies, the dying patient is more often than not psychologically isolated.[6] Among health care professionals, there is often a preference for treating the rare or challenging case. The emotionally supportive nursing care needed by an elderly, lingering, dying patient seems somehow to pale by comparison.[7]

Hospitals are not geared to create a homelike atmosphere, even though some of the newer and more modern institutions provide comforts approaching those of hotels. People's identities and sense of self are expressed in things such as home and possessions; they need to be able to control their own bodies and events directly affecting them. A few personal belongings come to represent security in the present through the past. To be forced to leave home and go into an institution even for a short period is difficult; it may be overwhelming when a prolonged period of time is involved.[8] Thus, patients' fears and despair can be almost overwhelming, and the understanding and consolation so sorely required are seldom available.

When most of us enter the hospital as patients, our roles require us to acquiesce to the physical probing, the exploration of our bodies, the sticking of needles, the ingesting of sometimes unpleasant-tasting and/or -smelling substances, the pushing, the pulling, the coughing, wheezing, grunting, groaning, and other indignities to which we may be exposed—all in the names of diagnosis and therapy. We expect our health to improve, the disease that brought us to this place somehow to be conquered. Even though we are grateful for the results when we are well on the road to recovery, we are annoyed at the time, because the hospital customs and procedures reflect that organizational efficiency has taken precedence over personal concern.

It is difficult in a busy hospital ward for the staff to give dying patients the understanding and the discriminating handling of drugs that they need for the relief of their symptoms. Their problems are different from those of the rest of the ward, and the staff are so hard-pressed by the demands of acute work that much relievable suffering is undoubtedly overlooked.[9] Nash, Connors, and Gemperle wrote that, "frequently the 'vacuum' of care received by the person in terminal illness erodes meaning and denies dignity."[10]

Hospitals or cancer centers may not always be the best place for cancer patients. They are not happy in the the midst of an open acute ward; they will probably know what such an admission means if they have been in the ward before, and their suffering will be intensified greatly by isolation. They find it trying to have major surgery and recovery going on all around them, and their presence may be disturbing to other patients as well as to the staff. Patients in separate or single rooms need extra staff if they are not to feel forgotten.[11] "As death becomes imminent, nursing care often is given less and less frequently," Mervyn informs us, and "when the dying patient becomes comatose, he is often treated as if he were, in fact, dead, for he is no longer communicating."[12]

The Closed Awareness Context

Frequently, hospitalized terminal patients do not fully understand the gravity of their conditions. Glaser and Strauss describe a "closed awareness context" wherein the hospital staff knows the patient is dying, but the patient is unaware. Most patients are not experienced at recognizing the signs of impending death, and the hospital is magnificently organized, both by accident and design, to hide the medical truth from patients. Records are kept out of reach. Medical talk about the patients generally occurs in far-removed places. Also, the staff is trained to act or is accustomed to acting collusively around patients, so as not to disclose medical secrets. The usual rationale for withholding information is, Why deny them all hope by telling them they are dying? Ordinarily, terminally ill patients have no allies who can help them discover staff secrets. Even their families or other patients will withhold such information if privy to it.[13] Essentially, there is a conspiracy of silence insulating the dying patient from the truth.

Intensive Care Units

Most modern general hospitals have an intensive care unit (ICU), a coronary care unit (CCU), or possibly a combination of the two—an intensive care/coronary unit (ICCU)—where the most advanced technological hardware and the most specially trained intensive care personnel (usually one RN to every two patients: a nursing ratio of 12 nursing hours per patient day) are available to attend to the most critical patients. Medical direction of the unit is provided by either a medical director, a panel of specialists, or a committee of the medical staff.

No matter the number of beds available in the unit, there will be times when all beds will be occupied with critically ill patients, and a new patient in critical condition is to be admitted. Take, for example, the case of a filled, six-bed CCU to which a seventh patient desperately needs to be admitted. There is no question that all seven patients need the specialized care offered by the unit or they will die. Yet only six can be accommodated. A medical decision needs to be made, and quickly. Which six of the seven will stay in this CCU? Which one will be sent to one of the nursing floors where the necessary technology and personnel skills may not be available? Can one, who may not survive the ambulance ride, be transferred to another hospital that may have an available CCU bed? How can the decision be explained to the family, or for that matter, to the patient who is rational and capable of understanding? In short, those charged with making such a medical decision sometimes have the awesome responsibility of playing God.

If one of those seven patients happens to have a terminal illness, the decision is somewhat less onerous, but still, physicians' training and scope of activity have been such that many physicians have ambivalent feelings about initiating passive euthanasia or discontinuing dysthanasia.

Family Needs

Most families want the patient to remain at home and eventually to die there. They feel that if the physician says that the patient needs to be admitted to the hospital, the act of going to the hospital is the first stage of dying.[14] Some relatives will see it as a failure on their part, and they need considerable reassurance from the physician that the admission was unavoidable.[15]

When seriously ill patients are brought to the ICU, CCU, or ICCU, the relatives will usually accompany them, but most hospitals do not have adequate facilities to accommodate the family. Families are usually left completely alone with no one to answer their questions or to talk with about their concerns. They spend their hours waiting in hallways, cafeterias, or anywhere around the hospital, walking aimlessly back and forth. Hospitals should have rooms adjacent to the intensive care units where relatives could sit, rest, and eat, where they could share their loneliness and perhaps console each other during the endless periods of waiting.[16] Social workers or chaplains should be available, with sufficient time for each relative; physicians and nurses should be frequent visitors to these "family rooms" to be available to talk and answer questions.[17]

Visiting Restrictions

All hospitals have visiting restrictions; hours may be from 10 A.M. to noon, 2 P.M. to 4 P.M., and 7 P.M. to 8 P.M. Such restrictions are not for the benefit of the patient, but for the staff's convenience, so that their duties can be efficiently discharged. In some hospitals, only two visitors are permitted at a time, theoretically to prevent the patient from becoming over-tired and to permit a turnover of visitors if more than two have come to see the patient. Yet some patients would thrive on more than two visitors at one time, while others may want only one, or none. Children under 14 years of age are generally not permitted to visit patients, supposedly because they are more susceptible to diseases or because they might transmit diseases to the patients—a moot point in the case of terminally ill patients.[18]

NURSING HOMES

In considering hospices for care of the terminally ill, Morris Kerstein writes that "the conversion of a nursing home or convalescent retreat [to a hospice facility] would be adequate neither as a physical or a psychological plant."[19] A high proportion of the patients in nursing homes are destined to die there or to be removed only at the very last minute for intensive hospital care, yet few of these institutions appear to have given much thought to the special problems of the dying.[20]

In many cases, it is quite difficult to get a patient into a nursing home. In Canada, a doctor must estimate that the patient has less than 60 days to live before many nursing homes will take the patient.[21] Parker Rossman points out the Catch-22 situation that exists between nursing homes and hospitals:

> The right sort of nursing home to take care of a terminally-ill person may not exist in a community. It was apparently the policy of the best nursing homes in the area not to accept terminally-ill people, and to send their own patients to hospitals when they became terminally ill. At the same time, the hospitals in the community had a policy of dismissing terminally-ill people in order to provide for persons who could be cured. To families who felt they could not take care of a dying patient at home, these hospitals recommended that they look for a nursing home! When this contradiction was pointed out to them, hospital and

> nursing home officials all expressed surprise at learning the policy of the other.[22]*

Many nursing homes are not pleasant places to visit, with odors lingering from incontinent patients and many senile, irrational patients creating a cacophony as one strolls through the corridors. Because of financial restrictions, the personnel tend to be poorly trained, which results in less-than-ideal conditions for care of the terminally ill patients. This is not meant to imply that all nursing homes fall into this category. There are numerous well-managed, well-maintained, bright nursing homes where patients are well cared for. However, specialized care for terminally ill patients is inadequate. In nursing homes, physicians need not be on duty every day, the pain-control philosophy of hospice care does not exist, and care of the patient and the family as a unit has not as yet been accepted.

At the Fourth Euthanasia Conference, the Reverend Cornelius Trowbridge discussed his nursing-home convalescence from an extended illness. He described the facility as a place where most of the patients had been put to die. He wrote, "The irony of the situation is that those places are the expression of our humanitarianism. The families who support them at great expense feel that they are doing all they can for their relatives." He added that he could see the virtuous look on the face of the daughter who would pay her weekly visit to her mother, who may or may not know that the daughter has been there.[23]

Reverend Trowbridge described the typical patients he observed in the nursing homes:

> It was the patients, the poor pathetic men and women in their wheelchairs who created an atmosphere that was utterly depressing. All but two of them were old, mainly in their eighties, some in their nineties. A few of them were mentally alert. The majority were senile or worse. They were fed, given their pills, taken to the bathroom, and then wheeled into the corridor where they sat slumped over in their chairs, until it was time to be fed again and finally put to bed and another day was over.[24]

This kind of existence does not begin to approach the humanitarian hospice concept. The patients described by Reverend Trowbridge may not be

---

*This and subsequent referenced citations reprinted by permission of the publisher from Parker Rossman, *Hospice: Creating New Models of Care for the Terminally Ill* (New York: Association Press, 1977). © 1977 by Association Press/Follett Publishing Co., 1010 W. Washington, Chicago, Illinois 60607.

much better off than Karen Ann Quinlan. The Reverend Trowbridge concluded his letter with, "Surely there can be no kindness or compassion in prolonging the life of someone in acute misery, such as the woman across the hall who kept up a continual wailing cry until she was mercifully sedated. Or another, whom I shall never forget who cried out at intervals, 'Oh, God, won't somebody help me?'"[25]

Nursing homes play a very important role in our modern health care delivery system. Unfortunately, unfavorable physical conditions and questionable practices of some of these institutions have received adverse publicity in the media in recent years. This has served to detract from the excellent character of service that is provided in most nursing homes for the chronically ill. However, the care of terminally ill patients should be left to those programs and institutions that offer specialized care of these patients, and not to the vagaries of a system that offers little more than small corners of the world that some describe as "vegetable bins."

COST CONSIDERATIONS

Dobihal feels strongly that hospice care is a system of care that offers a less expensive alternative to care that is now primarily based in acute general hospitals.[26] Kerstein feels that Medicare, Medicaid, and foundation support should be sufficient to reimburse hospice cost. Since elaborate testing and equipment would not be necessary for a hospice, he feels costs should be considerably lower than those for an acute-care hospital.[27]

Viola Reibe, an RN from Diablo Valley College, Contra Costa County, California, who spent five weeks working at St. Christopher's Hospice, London, stated that "overall hospice costs are generally lower than overall hospital costs because hospice is 'high on personnel, low on technology.'" (The latter quotation she attributes to Cicely Saunders of St. Christopher's Hospice.)[28] According to Elisabeth Kubler-Ross, when terminal patients are treated in hospitals, costs can run about $300 per day, but at home, using the Brompton cocktail for pain control, medication materials costs ran about 80¢ per week![29]

At this stage of hospice development, the matter of costs is an unresolved issue. Different views have been expressed by numerous people involved with the hospice movement. Few definitive studies have been performed to date. Judd says that "cost effectiveness must be addressed at two levels: (1) the comparative costs between conventional treatment and hospice treatment as a whole; and (2) a comparison of costs between models of hospice care."[30]

Proponents of free-standing hospice facilities contend that since the hospice facility does not have to finance expensive life-saving equipment, it does not have to amortize the cost of that technology by a charge against each occupied bed, and hence it can charge less per day. Take, for example, the high capital cost of hospital intensive care units, coronary care units, emergency departments, operating suites, labor and delivery units, hemodialysis units, cardiovascular stress laboratories, inhalation therapy and pulmonary function labs, diagnostic and therapeutic radiographic departments, clinical laboratories, and other expensive capital-intensive features of the modern hospital that are geared to cure the diseases of humanity. The proponents of separate hospice facilities claim that terminally ill patients should not have to pay for shares of the unneeded services and equipment. They also contend that if the hospice is located within a hospital facility, the very existence of such life-saving equipment and services could tempt some physicians to undertake "heroic measures" or to experiment with the dying patient by trying out new curative treatments.[31]

But let us not conclude that hospice care is cheap. On the contrary, operating costs are relatively high. In England, the per-patient cost is about 80 percent of that in a general hospital, and about 85 percent of the budget goes to staff salaries.[32] However, since a hospice facility needs only to have simple equipment and a homelike atmosphere,[33] its costs should be less than when a terminally ill patient is cared for in an acute-care general hospital.

While the hospice does not perform surgery, x-ray exams and many laboratory procedures, it does provide extensive and comprehensive nursing care. In the general hospital, nursing care is provided at the ratio of about 4.5 to 5.0 nursing hours per patient day. Stoddard claims that "nursing care . . . must be maintained at a far higher nurse-patient ratio than is found in hospitals and nursing homes."[34] As one study indicated, hospice inpatients require approximately nine hours of nursing care per patient day, not including volunteer assistance.[35] On a tight budget, one hospital's inpatient palliative care unit provides 6.5 to 7.0 nursing hours per patient day, but the unit director hastened to add that the ratio for "inpatient programs should be higher than this."[36]

The National Cancer Institute has reported that the average stay in hospice inpatient programs is from 13 to 18 days.[37] For 5,956 nonfederal, short-term general and other special hospitals, the average length of stay for 1976 was 7.7 days.[38] Thus, hospice inpatient stays are on the order of twice those of average acute general hospital patients who are hospitalized for cure of their diseases, but because capital-intensive costs are less and because ancillary services are kept at a minimum, overall costs per patient tend to be less for hospice patients than for acute general hospital patients.

The cost of home care has been estimated to be about 50 percent less than that of inpatient care, with outpatient care cost falling somewhere between. This has been translated by one hospice source as a potential savings to society of 7.4 *billion* dollars annually.[39]

NOTES

1. Florence Nightingale, *Notes on Hospitals,* 3rd ed. (London: Longman, Green, 1863), preface.
2. Melvin J. Krant, *Dying and Dignity: The Meaning and Control of a Personal Death* (Springfield, Illinois: Thomas, 1974), p. 58.
3. Frances Mervyn, "The Plight of Dying Patients in Hospitals," *American Journal of Nursing* 71 (October 1971): 1,988–90.
4. E. Mansell Pattison, *The Experience of Dying* (Englewood Cliffs, New Jersey: Prentice-Hall, 1977), p. 50.
5. Ibid.
6. Robert S. Morison, "Dying," *Life and Death and Medicine: A Scientific American Book* (San Francisco: W. H. Freeman, 1973), pp. 39–45.
7. Mervyn, loc. cit.
8. Krant, pp. 57–8.
9. Cicely Saunders, "The Need for In-Patient Care for the Patient with Terminal Cancer," *Middlesex Hospital Journal* 72 (February 1973).
10. Mary Louise Nash, Canice Connors, and Rosemary Gemperle, "Toward Dignity in Care: An In-Service Model," *Death Education* 1 (Spring 1977): 113–30.
11. Saunders, loc. cit.
12. Mervyn, loc. cit.
13. Barney Glaser and Anselm Strauss, "Awareness Contexts and Social Interaction," in *Death and Identity,* rev. ed., ed. Robert Fulton (Bowie, Maryland: Charles Press, 1976), pp. 144–58.
14. Richard Lamerton, *Care of the Dying* (Westport, Connecticut: Technomic Publishing Co., 1976), p. 33.
15. Ibid.
16. Elisabeth Kubler-Ross, *On Death and Dying* (New York: MacMillan, 1969), p. 147.
17. Ibid.
18. Ibid., p. 148.
19. Morris Kerstein, "Caring for the Terminally Ill: A Hospice," *American Journal of Psychiatry* 129 (August 1972): 237–8.
20. Morison, loc. cit.
21. Balfour Mount, "Death—A Part of Life?" *Crux* 11, no. 3 (1973–74): 3–6.
22. Parker Rossman, *Hospice: Creating New Models of Care for the Terminally Ill* (New York: Association Press, 1977), p. 52.

23. Cornelius Trowbridge, Letter appearing in *Dilemmas of Euthanasia: Excerpts from Papers and Discussion at the 4th Euthanasia Conference* (New York: The Euthanasia Educational Council, December 4, 1971), p. 27.

24. Ibid.

25. Ibid.

26. Edward T. Dobihal, Jr., "Talk or Terminal Care?" *Connecticut Medicine* 38 (July 1974): 364–7.

27. Morris D. Kerstein, "Caring for the Terminally Ill: A Hospice," *American Journal of Psychiatry* 129 (August 1972): 237–8.

28. Viola Riebe, in testimony at California Legislature, Assembly Committee on Health, Public Hearing on Hospices, Santa Barbara, California, December 1, 1977.

29. Elisabeth Kubler-Ross, "Living with Dying," Speech sponsored by Power Within, Lobero Theater, Santa Barbara, Calif., October 4, 1977.

30. Leda R. Judd, "Hospices—A Background Paper," Unpublished report prepared for HEW, n.d., p. 24.

31. Parker Rossman, *Hospice: Creating New Models of Care for the Terminally Ill* (New York: Association Press, 1977), p. 147.

32. C. Holden, "Hospices: For the Dying, Relief from Pain and Fear," *Science* 193 (July 30, 1976): 389–91.

33. Rossman, p. 210.

34. Sandol Stoddard, *The Hospice Movement: A Better Way of Caring for the Dying* (Briarcliff Manor, New York: Stein and Day, 1978), p. 170.

35. "The Hospice Movement," Unpublished Management Services Special Report (Newport Beach, California: Advanced Health Systems, Inc., 1977).

36. Janet Bauer, Director of the palliative care unit, Pinecrest Hospital, Santa Barbara, California, in testimony at California Legislature public hearing, loc. cit.

37. Letter from Lawrence D. Burke, Program Director for Rehabilitation Treatment, Rehabilitation and Continuing Care Branch (DCCR), National Cancer Institute, HEW, December 15, 1977.

38. *Hospital Statistics, 1977 Edition* (Chicago: American Hospital Association, 1977), Table 1, p. 4.

39. Advanced Health Systems report.

Chapter 8
Symptom Control

Those who do not feel pain seldom think that it is felt.
Samuel Johnson, *The Rambler*, no. 48

In the care of the terminally ill, by far the most critical symptom that must be relieved is pain. One can tell if a person is in pain simply by looking and listening. A wrinkled brow, tense fingers, and cautious breathing may betray underlying pain even in an unresponsive patient.[1] Not all suffering is pain, nor is all pain suffering, but the alleviation of suffering in patients with terminal illnesses, particularly cancer, is an important aspect of intervention.[2] No patients should want to die because of the pain they are suffering.[3]

THE FOUR TYPES OF PAIN

> When you are talking about controlling the pain of a terminal patient, you need to remember that it is not just a physical pain. By the time the patient has reached the terminal stages of his disease, he is suffering from many other types of pain, including mental, financial, interpersonal, and spiritual. You need to pay attention to the whole person if you are going to bring the physical complaints of pain under control.[4]

The four types of pain—social, psychological, spiritual, and physical—make up the total pain with which anyone caring for terminal patients must continually deal. The different types are so interwoven that it is very difficult to consider or treat them separately. To control this chronic pain successfully, the entire patient must be treated. All the aspects of pain must be understood and addressed before the pain can be brought under control. Since anxiety, depression, and insomnia can affect the patient's perception of pain, therapeutic activities and other distractions can help alleviate the pain. Once all the other components of pain have been identified, the physician can concentrate on the control of physical pain.[5]

Social Pain

> Social pain may be defined in two ways: (1) it may be defined as a patient's "mild-to-severe discomfort" with man's inhumanity to man—a common theme in the history of all technocratic civilizations, or (2) it may be defined as simply a patient's discomfort with the level and intensity of his or her interpersonal relationships, especially if one is in the process of dying . . . . [It is important] for the dying patient and his family to finish any unfinished interpersonal business including learning how to say goodby to one another for the last time.[6]

In dealing with social pain, the hospice facilitates *quality* social interaction. This helps patients live more fully until they die.

Physical pain naturally affects a person mentally. Anxiety can accompany breathlessness; depression can accompany nausea. The intense strain of trying to cope can be humiliating. Increasing helplessness and dependency are difficult burdens, but the care givers, particularly nurses, can help patients understand that their value as people has not diminished as a result of their situations.

Patients need someone to listen to them, to share their loneliness and fears. Panic attacks and demands for attention will cease when patients realize that the care givers are nearby, that they care, and that they will not leave the patients alone.

Maintaining some sort of social life up to the end is vital for terminal patients, because facing the unknown alone and friendless is frightening to contemplate. The care givers, other patients, patients' families, and volunteers all contribute to this social life by sharing some of the pain. Talk is therapeutic and can prepare patients and their families for the inevitable. By preventing social pain from taking over, the care giver provides additional opportunities for the grieving process to begin before the patient dies.[7] Thus, the patient and the family are eased into anticipatory grief which is a transition for both the patient and the loved ones.

Psychological Pain

> The dying patient experiencing "psychological pain" is frequently the frightened or anxious patient, the lonely or de-

> pressed patient, or the hurt and angry patient. As he begins his final stage of growth by anticipating his own mortality, the terminally ill patient often endeavors to "set things in balance" by attempting to maintain a kind of psychological homeostasis of equi-finality with his inner self and *his* perceptions of the immediate environment. This imbalance or loss of control over his or her life, especially the now "new" experience of learning how to die, usually calls up a repertoire of coping behaviors aimed chiefly at reducing the stresses of dying and at regaining control over one's life . . . . Thirty minutes of cathartic grieving with a family member, nurse, or skilled therapist can have profound positive effects on a dying patient's depression and concomitant anxiety.[8]

A woman in severe pain with spinal metastases from breast cancer was hospitalized six weeks before telling the orderly that her greatest fear about having cancer was that the malignancy would spread upwards and that she would die, like a leper, with tumors all over her face. The usual drug program during that six weeks did not relieve the pain; the underlying anxiety caused her pain to continue. After she had expressed her fears to the orderly, the doctor spoke to her about the fact that it just wasn't going to happen. When her psychological and physical symptoms were both controlled, her pain disappeared and she went home.[9]

Spiritual Pain

Woodson has said that, "to date there is no clear-cut definition of what constitutes 'spiritual pain,' particularly as it relates to the dying. Spiritual pain is as different for each patient as is the patient's specific religious, transracial, or cultural background."[10] Yet spiritual pain does exist, and though it manifests itself differently in each patient, the deep internal, subjective, endopsychic feelings can be relieved by counseling with trained clergy or other counselors.

Physical Pain

By far the most debilitating of the four kinds of pain is physical pain. There are two kinds of physical pain: acute and chronic. Physicians are well trained in treating acute pain, but they are untrained in treating chronic pain.[11] Pain management is really the key to good hospice care; after pain management is accomplished, other symptoms can be more easily managed.[12] In Walter Norman's opinion, "our major concern has to be focused on the control of pain rather than the alleviation of pain."[13] For the cancer patient, in particular, pain has a sinister meaning.[14] Most people who awake in the morning with a stiff neck assume that they left a window open and slept in a draft. Cancer patients who wake with a stiff neck assume that the malignancy is spreading. The degree of pain is perceived totally differently in these two situations.[15]

Cancer pain is protopathic; that is, it is constant, persistent—the chronic pain of terminal disease, without meaning or purpose. It gets worse rather than better, and it is a very different thing from the acute pains of normal life that all doctors and patients are fully aware of from personal experience.[16]

Physical pain is that constant or occasional discomfort ranging from a mild toothache to severe and chronic debilitating pain of the advanced-stage cancer patient.[17] "Acute pain is reversible. It warns us of a problem that needs attention. It can therefore be viewed as linear, with a beginning and an end. Chronic pain, however, can be characterized as a vicious circle with no set time limit."[18] Pain is "not simply a matter of electrical impulses travelling up particular nerves . . . . Long-standing relentless pain is almost a disease in itself, because of the devastating effects it has on the person. He cannot get away from it, it commands his attention, and yet it seems completely meaningless."[19]

PAIN CONTROL THROUGH DRUGS

Cicely Saunders has written that in British hospices, 70 percent of the patients have pain that must be controlled with narcotics.[20] Sylvia Lack, medical director of Hospice, Inc., said that not all cancer patients develop pain, that only 40 percent suffer moderate to severe pain.[21] And Parker Rossman claims that, "of fifteen hundred British hospice patients, 99 percent arrived at the hospice in severe pain."[22] Even though these three authorities disagree on the percentages of hospice and/or cancer patients who have severe pain, the fact remains that the control of pain in cancer patients is a problem of huge dimensions.

As Richard Lamerton has observed, "Most people can cope with short term pain, but what we most fear is pain which lasts for months."[23] As opposed to the acute pain of headache, where the medication for relief is given after the fact, the unremitting pain in terminal cancer requires that the treatment regimen *prevent* pain rather than attempt to control it once it is present.[24] "If pain is properly controlled," as it is in a hospice, "the patient will never feel it again."[25]

> At the heart of the hospice concept is a view of pain control which runs counter to the way a general hospital nurse is

> taught—i.e., to withhold pain medicine until the patient demands it—or the hospital procedure by which a patient is given pain medicine on a fixed routine of every four hours even though he or she may begin to suffer serious pain within three hours. The [hospice] staff . . . assume that once it is definite that a person is dying, then the comfort of the patient takes precedence. Instead of waiting until a patient is miserable with pain to give relief, instead of waiting for the patient to demand the medicine because of his or her suffering, the hospice staff anticipates pain and gives the drug before the pain occurs, so that the patient never experiences any serious pain at all.[26]

For the dying, there is no maximum dose of a pain killer. If, because a tolerance has built up, a patient requires five times the normal dosage, then that is the correct dosage.[27] Proper drug management for the dying is definitely not the PRN (as the occasion arises, as needed) order for pain medication that is seen in the acute-care hospital. The patient in a PRN regimen has to be in severe pain before getting relief, which causes a cycle of pain, anxiety, suffering, and depression, the anticipation of which triggers even more severe pain.

> The expectation of pain produces anxiety which in turn, compounds the pain. The patient who is confident he will be as pain-free as possible will be more at ease and may in the end require less rather than more medication. To the traditional physician, this is an unaccustomed approach. Physicians are afraid to addict the patient; that is what they learned in medical school and their reaction is to underprescribe.[28]

In hospices, however, minimally sufficient drugs are ordered frequently enough to hold pain in abeyance.[29]

Narcotics are especially useful for the relief of intense pain; they are the most effective analgesics known. The term *narcotic*, in current usage, means opium, its derivatives, or synthetic substitutes that produce tolerance and dependence, both psychological and physical. Narcotics may create a short-lived state of euphoria. They also tend to induce drowsiness, apathy, lethargy, decreased physical activity, constipation, pinpoint pupils, and reduced vision. Larger doses may induce sleep, nausea, vomiting, and respiratory depression—the major toxic effect of the opiates.[30]

Some physicians feel that larger doses of narcotics, because of their inhibitory effect on breathing, may shorten patients' lives. Others' experience has been quite the opposite. They have found that by easing the sense of breathlessness as well as the pain, those drugs relieve the distress that can exhaust the dying. Being able to rest, they live longer.[31]

Experimental Drugs

The issue of new, experimental drugs for the fatally ill is a thorny one. Patients should have reasonably good chances to benefit from the drug in spite of its unpleasant or possibly life-shortening effects, e.g., hair loss, blistering of mouth, nausea, vomiting, and skin rashes.[32] In the case of terminally ill patients who are in great pain, the loss of individuality that may come from massive doses of pain killers may be seen as more humane than the loss of individuality through unbearable suffering, even though the treatment for pain may also hasten the patient's death.[33]

Heroin and Morphine

Most American doctors describe narcotics as "bad medicine" because they make people addicts. When a person is in perpetual, agonizing pain and has only a few weeks to live, that's pretty much a moot point. Heroin is an excellent pain killer. It makes patients calmer and causes less nausea and vomiting than morphine. Morphine is not banned in the United States, but heroin, its derivative, is. American and Canadian physicians noted that an irrational fear of narcotics, spawned by the specter of drug addiction in society at large, has left many doctors unwilling to provide effective pain control.[34]

David Trebach of the American University Law School in Washington, D.C., argues, "There's no rational reason why heroin shouldn't be made available for medical use because it's one of the greatest pain killers we have. The World Health Organization lists 38 countries that allow heroin for medical reasons. It's obscene that we do not have it."[35] The fight to legalize heroin for medical use in the United States has been spearheaded by the National Committee on the Treatment of Intractable Pain (Judith Quattlebaum, President, P.O. Box 34571, Washington, D.C. 20034). Peter Bourne, former special assistant to President Jimmy Carter, called for the National Institutes of Health to reassess drugs such as heroin and marijuana for possible use in alleviating terminal pain.[36] In January 1978, Representative Neil Abercrombie of Hawaii introduced House Concurrent Resolution No. 16, which is a request to the United States attorney general to allow the use of heroin for medical purposes. In May 1978, Assembly Bill No. A. 12078 and Senate Bill No. S. 9098 were introduced into the New York state legislature, both bills providing that doctors be allowed to administer controlled substances, such as heroin and marijuana, to patients who are terminally ill. On April 27, 1978, Commissioner Norbert Wisniewski introduced a resolution, passed by the Board of Commissioners of Wayne County, Michigan, supporting the medical profession's use of otherwise illegal drugs that have shown proven medicinal value; safeguards would, of course, be enacted to guard against unlawful distribution.

In March 1978, a heroin resolution was adopted by the Commission on Social Action Reform Judaism (the Union of American Hebrew Congregations in conjunction with the Central Conference of American Rabbis). The resolution urges the United States attorney general to remove heroin from Drug Schedule I of the Controlled Substances Act, which designates it of no medical use, to Schedule II, which places it in the same restricted category as morphine.[37] The attorney general has the authority, under the Comprehensive Drug Abuse Prevention and Control Act of 1970 (P.L. 91-513), to make this transfer.

In a January 1978 address to the National Committee on the Treatment of Intractable Pain, Robert Twycross startled the hospice community with the following statement:

> When given intravenously, diamorphine [heroin] has an earlier onset of action, is more sedative, and causes less vomiting than morphine. These are all properties which are desirable when seeking to relieve severe, acute pain. By mouth, because diamorphine is metabolized in the gut and by the liver, there is no real difference between orally administered diamorphine and orally administered morphine, in terms of analgesic effect and other actions . . . .
>
> When injections are necessary, diamorphine is undoubtedly the best and safest of all the potent narcotic analgesics and is indispensable in the care of a proportion of patients with advanced cancer.[38]

In a 1965 article, Cicely Saunders, founder and medical director of St. Christopher's Hospice in Sydenham, London wrote, "We use this drug [heroin] almost exclusively. We have found that although the other opiates . . . may relieve pain just as effectively, only [heroin] will do so with so few side effects or leave the patients so alert and serene."[39] St. Christopher's annual report for 1976–1977, however, reported that since nearly all the doses of analgesics are administered orally, morphine is now the narcotic of choice at St. Christopher's Hospice, even though diamorphine, with its greater solubility, is used for rare parenteral (extraintestinal) use.[40]

Lysergic Acid Diethylamide (LSD)

The psychedelic drug, LSD (lysergic acid diethylamide), has been used by researchers in pain relief, but was withdrawn about 10 years ago by federal regulations. Psychiatrist Eric C. Kast has reported using it successfully on 90 terminal patients. A precipitous drop in pain occurs in two or three hours after LSD administration. This relief lasts about 12 hours, and the total pain intensity diminishes for about three weeks, after which the body may build up a tolerance to the drug.[41]

Brompton's Cocktail

A potent oral analgesic mixture that is used to relieve and prevent the pain associated with selected cases of terminal cancer is called Brompton's Cocktail, Brompton Mixture or Hospice Mix. The standard mixture contains a variable amount of morphine or diamorphine (heroin, in countries other than the United States), 10 mg. of cocaine, 2.5 ml. of ethyl alcohol (98 percent), 5 ml. of flavoring syrup, and a variable amount of chloroform water, for a total of 20 ml.[42] Hospice, Inc. in New Haven, Connecticut uses morphine dissolved in cherry syrup combined with a phenothiazine in their Hospice Mixture. Sylvia Lack, medical director, claims that they do not use cocaine, alcohol, or chloroform water because they are not necessary for good pain control.[43]

Brompton's Cocktail should be given in 20-ml. doses with phenothiazine every four hours around the clock because the serum half-life of morphine taken orally is about four hours.[44] Because it is generally given every four hours in the attempt to maintain continuous control over pain, this therapy also diminishes the fear or expectation of pain, thereby decreasing pain still further.

Using the McGill-Melzack pain questionnaire, Melzack, Ofiesh, and Mount conducted a study of 92 patients at the Royal Victoria Hospital in Montreal. The study showed that the Brompton Cocktail controlled pain in 90 percent of the patients in the palliative care unit and 75 to 80 percent of the patients in wards or private rooms. The Brompton Cocktail provides a powerful tool for the control of pain in most patients with cancer. Moreover, it does not act on only a single dimension of pain, but has a strong effect on the physical, emotional, and psychological dimensions together.[45]

Lack indicates that one of the reasons why she gives narcotics as an oral liquid is because the dosage of a liquid may be titrated more finely than it can be with tablets. Titration, the estimation of a drug's concentration, is necessary to find the dose that controls the pain but doesn't sedate the patient. This dosage may be within a very fine range.[46]

The Brompton Mixture, to be effective against the total pain of advanced malignant disease, must be used in combination with other therapies. Symptom control may require additional measures such as radiotherapy, peripheral nerve or intrathecal block, neurosurgery, or physical measures such as splinting and passive exercises.[47]

RELIEF OF SECONDARY SYMPTOMS

Dying patients may have numerous minor ailments in addition to those symptoms directly associated with terminal illnesses—loss of appetite, nausea and vomiting, hiccups, itching, labored breathing, coughing, insomnia, depression, anxiety, incontinence, constipation, and difficulty in swallowing. All of these need to be attended to and not allowed to cause discomfort. The symptoms of dehydration, for example, are usually combatted by frequent mouth washes and vaseline on the lips.[48] The dehydrated patient should not be stabbed with intravenous needles; a drink to sip or a bit of crushed ice to suck may be just as effective and much easier on a wasted body.[49]

Of all patients administered narcotics for pain control, 100 percent will develop constipation,[50] which is not only uncomfortable, but may also have serious consequences if not relieved. Surprisingly, it is the minor symptoms that can sometimes distress the patient the most. Loss of appetite may be causing more immediate concern than the bone cancer; having hiccups may at the time seem more burdensome than having a tumor. To improve the quality of life for terminally ill patients, the care givers must take an intense interest in and be experts in total symptom control.

SUMMARY

While terminally ill patients suffer from many symptoms, both primary and secondary, and from several different types of pain, the most critical symptom that must be controlled is chronic physical pain. Narcotics, regularly administered, are the most effective means of controlling this pain. Taken in regular doses, a narcotic can be used for many months without the need to escalate the dose. Psychological dependence is created when the medication is *not* given in adequate doses on a regular basis.[51] The aim is to make the patient free of pain, by arranging for the continuous dosages of analgesics to be given so that the patient is always one step ahead of the pain. When a patient's fears and anxieties are relieved, the dosages can often be lowered, because so much of the subjective sensation of pain comes from emotional distress.[52]

It is just as important to decide when medication is no longer necessary, or when reduced amounts are required, as it is to prescribe more analgesics in larger amounts.[53] "In the last 48 hours of a patient's life, when toxicity has increased, circulation is stagnant, and excretion low," Lipman tells us that, "the patient may be just as comfortable and more alert with less medication, and there can be meaningful moments with loved ones until the very end."[54] Too much medication can prevent such opportunities.

Cicely Saunders says that better pain control in hospitals would make many admissions to her hospice unnecessary.[55] Inadequate pain control in hospitals is attributable partly to doctors' pharmacological ignorance and partly to the belief that analgesics should be administered sparingly to prevent the patient from becoming addicted and to avoid damaging side effects—considerations that are irrelevant to the dying. When the principles of pain control that are appropriate for the curable are also applied to the terminally ill, the result is often appallingly inhumane.

NOTES

1. Richard Lamerton, *Care of the Dying* (Westport, Connecticut: Technomic Publishing Co., 1976), p. 46.
2. Joan Craven and Florence S. Wald, "Hospice Care for Dying Patients," *American Journal of Nursing* 75 (October 1975): 1,816–22.
3. Sylvia Lack, Private Instruction Sheet Prepared by Medical Director, Hospice, Inc., New Haven, Connecticut, n.d., mimeographed.
4. Sylvia Lack, "I Want To Die While I'm Still Alive," *Death Education* 1, no. 2 (Summer 1977: 165–76.
5. Lack, Private Instruction Sheet.
6. Robert Woodson, "The Concept of Hospice Care in Terminal Disease," *Breast Cancer*, J. M. Vaeth, ed. (Basel, Switzerland: Karger, 1976): 161–79.
7. Ibid.
8. Ibid.
9. Lack, "I Want to Die," loc. cit.
10. Woodson, loc. cit.
11. William M. Lamers, in testimony at California Legislature, Assembly Committee on Health, Public Hearing on Hospice, Santa Barbara, California, December 1, 1977.
12. "Hospice," Interview with William M. Lamers, Medical Director, Hospice of Marin, *Thanatos*, March 1977, pp. 6–11.
13. Norman T. Walter, "The Coming of Death in America: Concepts in Transition," mimeographed, July 15, 1976, p. 14.
14. Lack, "I Want To Die," loc. cit.

15. Ibid.

16. T. S. West, "Hospice Care for a Dying Person and His Family," (Paper given at the First International Conference on Patient Counselling, Amsterdam, April 1976).

17. Woodson, loc. cit.

18. B. M. Mount et al., "Use of the Brompton Mixture in Treating the Chronic Pain of Malignant Disease," *Canadian Medical Association Journal* 115 (July 17, 1976): 122–4.

19. Lamerton, p. 107.

20. Cicely Saunders, "The Need for In-Patient Care for the Patient with Terminal Cancer," *Middlesex Hospital Journal* 72 (February 1973).

21. Lack, "I Want To Die," loc. cit.

22. Parker Rossman, *Hospice: Creating New Models of Care for the Terminally Ill* (New York: Association Press, 1977), p. 89.

23. Lamerton, p. 47.

24. Craven and Wald, loc. cit.

25. Lamerton, p. 106.

26. Rossman, p. 89.

27. Lamerton, p. 47.

28. Alice Kantor, "Focus on Hospice: Improving the Quality of Life That Remains," *St Luke's Hospital Center News* New York, n.d., pp. 3–4.

29. Walter, p. 18.

30. Federal Drug Enforcement Administration, *Drugs of Abuse* (Washington, D.C.: U.S. Government Printing Office, n.d.), p. 2.

31. Lamerton, p. 47.

32. Melvin J. Krant, *Dying and Dignity: The Meaning and Control of a Personal Death* (Springfield, Illinois: Charles Thomas, 1974), p. 63.

33. Jay Katz and Alexander M. Capron, *Catastrophic Diseases: Who Decides What?* (New York: Russell Sage Foundation, 1975), p. 26.

34. Michael Satchell, "How to Enjoy Life—Up to the Last Moment," *Parade,* October 16, 1977.

35. Ibid., citing Trebach.

36. *Newsletter of the National Committee on the Treatment of Intractable Pain* 1, no. 1 (Washington, D.C., January 1978): 1.

37. *Newsletter of the National Committee on the Treatment of Intractable Pain* 1, no. 4 (Washington, D.C., June 1978): 4.

38. Robert G. Twycross, "Address to the National Committee on the Treatment of Intractable Pain, January 31, 1978, Washington, D.C.," *Newsletter of the National Committee on the Treatment of Intractable Pain* 1, no. 2 (Washington, D.C., March 1978): 1–2.

39. Cicely Saunders, "The Last Stages of Life," *American Journal of Nursing* 65 (March 1965): 70–5.

40. St. Christopher's Hospice, "Annual Report, 1976–77," p. 16.

41. Arthur J. Snider, "LSD for the Terminally Ill?" *Los Angeles Times,* May 12, 1978, part IV, pp. 8–9.

42. Mount et al., loc. cit.

43. Lack, Private Instruction Sheet.

44. Mount et al., loc. cit.

45. R. Melzack, J. G. Ofiesh and B. M. Mount, "The Brompton Mixture: Effects on Pain in Cancer Patients," *Canadian Medical Association Journal* 115 (July 17, 1976): 125–8.

46. Lack, "I Want To Die," loc. cit.

47. Mount et al., loc. cit.

48. Lack, "I Want To Die," loc. cit.

49. William Hines, "London Hospice Dedicated to Serving the Terminally Ill," *Los Angeles Times,* December 9, 1977.

50. William M. Lamers, "Hospice Care—A New Concept for the Care of the Terminally Ill and Their Families," paper delivered at UCLA Extension Workshop, Los Angeles, California, April 8–9, 1978.

51. Lack, Private Instruction Sheet.

52. C. Holden, "Hospices: for the Dying, Relief from Pain & Fear," *Science* 193 (July 30, 1976): 389–91.

53. Craven and Wald, loc. cit.

54. A. C. Lipman, "Drug Therapy in Terminally Ill Patients," *American Journal of Hospital Pharmacy* 32 (March 1975): 270–6.

55. Holden, citing Saunders, loc. cit.

Chapter 9

Reimbursement

Too little payment for so great a debt.
Shakespeare, *The Taming of the Shrew*

Third-party reimbursement is crucial to hospice development—truly, to its survival. Today, more than 95 percent of the population is covered by some form of health insurance.[1] This includes both government (federal, state, local) programs and private insurance companies.

At present, laws governing reimbursement policies discriminate against the dying by providing funding for cure, not care.[2] The reimbursement policies of third-party payers must be changed; this means that laws must also be changed. Rossman quotes one physician who said:

> "A separate facility might be ideal, but we must at present keep our terminally-ill patients scattered all over the hospital to hide from Federal authorities the fact that we are accepting funds for their care to which we are not technically entitled." Another physician related to a hospice program at a hospital said: "We have to lie a little by not making it clear in our records that Patient X is terminally ill. Otherwise Blue Cross or his insurance company would not pay full rates. They would insist, rather, that the patient be dismissed from the hospital if he or she can no longer be cured."[3]

The central theme of hospices, that the patient and the family are the unit of care, is foreign to all third-party payers. Therefore, reimbursement does not provide for bereavement care or many of the social work functions of a hospice home care program.[4] The hospice approach of transfer from the home to an institution as the patient's condition changes, runs counter to Medicare regulations, which require that admission to a skilled nursing facility be preceded by a three-day hospital stay. Even if patients were transferred from home to hospital to hospice, many hospice facilities are not classified as skilled nursing facilities.

Because quality can follow closely in the footsteps of reimbursement, less reimbursement for a terminal-care bed than for an acute-care bed could conceivably mean a continued low priority for hospital-based hospice care.[5]

A group of hospice advocates, in negotiating with one hospital, ran into a Catch 22 due to the undecided role of insurance companies, Medicare, and Medicaid.

- The hospital wanted assurances that insurance companies would pay for the care before it would commit itself to leasing the beds.
- Insurance companies wanted promises that the facility would be licensed.
- The state health department wanted to know what its operating cost would be before it would grant a license. The discussion is further complicated because, as far as regulations and the law goes, a hospice hangs somewhere between a hospital and a nursing home, fitting into neither category.[6]

The issue of reimbursement is tied closely to that of licensing—a state function. Most states provide for licensing and inspection of all clinics, hospitals, skilled nursing facilities, and intermediate-care facilities. Some states require licensing of home health agencies, while others are considering licensing such agencies. Numerous regulations governing the safety and welfare of patients, visitors, and personnel are prescribed. Many conditions must be met in order to receive either state or federal funds. Those regulations are very specific for the facilities and agencies that are licensed; however, since hospices seem to be a type of hybrid, they are neither licensed by the states nor recognized by the federal government for reimbursement purposes.

Generally, functioning inpatient hospices are being reimbursed for some hospice services since they are licensed as acute general hospitals. In most cases, however, reimbursement is not provided for such hospice services as hospital-based home care services, counseling services for both patient and family, and bereavement follow-up services.

As mentioned previously, patients are accepted into Hospice, Inc. in New Haven, Connecticut, on the basis of health care need, not on ability to pay.[7] No British hospice discriminates against patients because of their financial status, and many feel that American hospices must also strive to uphold this altruistic approach. Most of the hospices in Britain are not under the National Health Service but are financed by a combination of charitable donations, patient contributions, and government reimbursement.[8]

According to a recent news item appearing in *Modern Healthcare,* Hospice, Inc. will receive reimbursement through Blue Cross-Blue Shield of Connecticut for hospice care and treatment. Services such as home visits and speech, hearing, dietary, and drug therapy will be reimbursed under the plan's home health care program. When the 44-bed facility now under construction opens, inpatient benefits will be provided.[9]

William Lamers, medical director of Hospice of Marin in Kentfield, California, testified at a public hearing of the California Assembly Health Committee that he feels reimbursement should be made on a lump-sum-per-case rather than fee-for-service basis. He feels that this approach would be simpler to administer; more easily understood by patients, families, doctors, and third-party payers; more equitable; and easy to determine and adjust with experience gained.[10]

The real problem may well be the fact that those who should be informed about hospice care of terminally ill patients, such as insurance company decision makers and legislators, are ill informed. As a result, most terminally ill are already ruled out by existing law, or defined out by institutional policy. More and more people are feeling that better care for less can be provided for more people at home, but for the terminally ill, this will mean changes in the law.[11]

INSURANCE COMPANY SURVEY

Background research for this work included a survey conducted to determine the extent to which private insurance companies have knowledge of hospices and to determine to what extent they recognize hospices by virtue of the hospice benefits they provide in their health insurance plans. Since some of the insurance companies are fiscal intermediaries for the Medicare program, an attempt was also made to determine to what extent the federal government of the United States recognizes the hospice movement by paying providers for hospice services through the Medicare program. Comments and suggestions from the insurance carriers were encouraged.

Although hospices are relatively new to the North American health care scene, they have been functioning for many years in Great Britain. Reimbursement philosophies for health care services in Great Britain and the United States are considerably different. In Great Britain, the bulk of health care service payments to providers comes from charitable donations, patient contributions, and government reimbursement.[12] By contrast, in the United States payment for health care in 1971 was 63 percent from third parties (public funds and private insurance benefits) and 37 percent from direct payments by the consumer.[13]

About 3,000 insurance companies in the United States write health and medical insurance.[14] However, only about 600 of these companies, all of which are listed in Francis B. Kelly's *1977-1978 Nationwide Hospital Insurance Billing Directory,* sell approximately 96 percent of the health insurance in the United States.[15]

Prior research has revealed that third-party payment practices for hospice benefits, except in a few isolated instances, do not exist. Because nearly two-thirds of all health care payments originate with third parties, future hospice development could depend upon their payment practices.

Methodology

Although personal or telephone interviews of the nearly 600 selected insurance companies in the United States, Canada, and Puerto Rico would have yielded the most reliable information, a mail survey was decided upon as the most practical method of collecting the necessary data. If properly designed, a questionnaire can be quite valuable. Even so, according to Selltiz et al., mailed questionnaire responses are usually low, varying from about 10 to 50 percent.[16] Despite the biases inherent in the method selected, a simple one-page questionnaire and letter of transmittal (see Appendices C and D) were designed. Each letter was addressed to the vice president, Group and Individual Health Services, of each insurance company.

Because of the limitations and potential biases inherent in the mail questionnaire method, readers are cautioned not to assume that these results represent all the insurance companies, since some did not respond. This survey is not to be considered as a statistically valid sampling of all insurance companies. The results should be viewed only as possible indicators of practices of some of the insurance carriers.

Results

A total of 582 questionnaires were mailed; 145 responses were received, for a total response rate of 25 percent (see Table 9-1). Since anonymity was assured, no insurance companies are identified except where permission was specifically granted.

The 403 independent insurance companies surveyed were identified in Kelly[17] as writers of accident and health insurance, but not all companies write major medical coverage. According to Kelly, the 47 fleets of companies represented 419 aggregate companies.[18] The 132 Blue Cross and Blue Shield plans are herewith simply identified as Blues.

Table 9-1 Summary of Responses to Insurance Company Survey

	Mailing	Responses Number	%
Independent Insurance Companies	403	97	24
Fleets or Groups of Companies	47	12	26
Blues	132	36	27
Totals	582	145	25

Of the 145 responses, 15 replied that they no longer write health insurance, and one indicated no desire to respond, yielding 129 net responses (see Table 9-2).

Question 1

Does your company represent a fleet or group of insurance companies? If yes, how many insurance companies does it represent?

This question does not apply to the independent companies. Of the 12 companies identified in Kelly as fleets, 11 responded with the number of insurance companies they represent. The twelfth fleet company responded with an informational letter only but did not indicate the number of insurance companies it represents; however, the count in Kelly's is assumed here as the correct count (see Table 9-3). The 12 fleet companies represent 88 individual insurance companies. Of the 36 responses from the Blues, four indicated they represent a fleet or group of insurance companies (see Table 9-4).

Table 9-2 Summary of Net Responses to Insurance Company Survey

	Independents	Fleets	Blues	Total
Responses	97	12	36	145
No longer write health insurance or no desire to respond	14	2	0	16
Net responses	83	10	36	129

Table 9-3 Number of Insurance Companies Represented by the 12 Fleets

Fleet Company	Insurance Companies Represented	Fleet Company	Insurance Companies Represented
A	4	G	40
B	5	H	3
C	3	I	6
D	3	J	2
E	7	K	5
F	3	L	7

The 145 total responses, therefore, represent a grand total of 363 insurance companies. Because of the format presented in Kelly, however, it is not clear if the additional count of 218 companies (363–145) were in part included in the separate 145 responses received, or if all of them are additional to the 145. Because of this unresolved point, the balance of this section will be concerned with only the 145 gross and the 129 net responses. It seems probable, however, that on the order of 50–150 additional companies above the 129 are represented due to the nonquantifiable number of individual companies represented by the fleets.

Question 2

Is your company or are any companies in the fleet a Medicare fiscal intermediary?

Table 9-4 Number of Insurance Companies Represented by Blue Fleets

Blue Fleet Company	Insurance Companies Represented
M	70
N	2
O	2
P	72
Total	146

Of the total net responses (129), 36—or 28 percent—indicated they are Medicare fiscal intermediaries (MFIs). Two percent of the independents, 10 percent of the fleets, and 92 percent of the Blues indicated that they are MFIs (see Table 9-5).

Question 3

Do any of your accident and health plans, group or individual, provide hospice benefits in the following form? (Check all that apply.)

Since a respondent could check one or more boxes, Lines a through f are not additive. (See Table 9-6.) However, by subtracting the sum of line g and "No response" from the totals of the net responses, we can arrive at the number of insurance companies that do provide hospice benefits and the number that do not (see Table 9-7).

Only 22 (17 percent) of the companies provide benefits, while the overwhelming majority, 107 (83 percent) of the net respondents do not provide hospice benefits.

Question 4

If you provide hospice benefits, what limitations, if any, do your plans impose?

Since this was a question requiring write-in answers, some respondents qualified their answers to Question 3 while others made general comments. Following are the most pertinent replies.

Table 9-5 Is your company or are any companies in the fleet a Medicare fiscal intermediary?

	Independents	Fleets	Blues	Total
Yes	2	1	33	36
No	79	9	2	90
Uncertain	1	0	1	2
No response	1	0	0	1

Table 9-6 Do any of your accident and health plans, group or individual, provide hospice benefits in the following form?

	Independents	Fleets	Blues	Total
a. As separate hospice facility	1	1	1	3
b. As separate department of general hospital	9	3	3	15
c. As home care hospice services	5	1	2	8
d. A multidisciplinary team which provides services wherever patient is located in hospital	4	2	1	7
e. Outpatient clinic hospice services	3	1	0	4
f. Other (please specify)	7	3	1	11
g. None of the above	66	5	28	99
h. No response	5	1	2	8

Independents

A Utah-based company stated, "In Arizona only—licensed home health agencies—Medicare supplements—20 percent of charges." Another company wrote, "We provide benefits for medical services only which are required to treat the condition." A third company answered,

Table 9-7 Insurance Companies Providing/Not Providing Hospice Benefits

	Independents	Fleets	Blues	Total
Total net responses	83	10	36	129
Insurance companies providing benefits	12	4	6	22
Insurance companies not providing benefits	71	6	30	107

"Covered services under major medical policies. Eligible expenses as enumerated under specific contracts."

One company that said it provides all services added the following qualification: "Our contract provides medically necessary treatment—in a hospital fitting our definition. Counselling is not medically necessary and probably would not be covered. Medically necessary and hospital definition control."

A company that sells daily hospital benefits only, no miscellaneous benefits included, wrote, "Half benefits in a convalescent home, which is qualified according to the terms of the policy, up to 100 days."

A company that checked 3b (separate hospital department) and added, "(if there are any?)" commented, "Not aware of any hospices currently operating in this country. Our plans generally do not cover persons over 65." A company that answered 3b (separate hospital department) with "Yes" and 3c (home care), d (multidisciplinary teams), and e (outpatient) as "?" responded with, "Hospice benefits as a defined policy benefit are not provided under any of our policies."

A company that answered 3b (hospital dept.), c (home care), d (multidisciplinary team), and e (outpatient) as "Some" added, "Our plans do not provide specific benefits for hospice services, but we do cover some of the services furnished by a hospice under our basic, major medical or comprehensive plans."

One company wrote, "Our group plan . . . will pay for general nursing care during confinement in a nursing home which subsequently follows a period of hospital confinement up to a maximum of 90 days during a calendar year." Another bluntly wrote, "Generally we would not pay for custodial care of a terminally ill patient." Still another company commented on services checked in 3b (hospital department), d (multidisciplinary team), and f (other), "If in an extended care facility approved by Medicare, provided confinement is not primarily custodial, and provided charges are billed in the name of *the hospital.*"

One company commented on 3f (other), "Certain types of 'care,' to the patient, only, by a qualified visiting nurse, might be a covered expense." A New England company commented that they provide home care hospice services under "statutory limits in accord with state requirements." A southwestern company added after home care services, "physicians or nurses only."

Finally, a midwestern company commented that, "We haven't encountered 3b above (separate hospital department) and would need more facts; we don't know what is meant by 3d (multidisciplinary team)."

Fleets

A southwestern group of 40 companies qualified 3f (other) with, "Our contracts pay for the services of RNs and MDs under major medical." A midwestern fleet of three companies that checked 3b (hospital department), and d (multidisciplinary team) explained, "Only if provided by doctor or other permitted dispenser of services. Also pays for inpatient hospital, etc." A New England group of three companies added after 3f (other), "Covers medical services while in general hospital." A different New England fleet of seven companies checked 3b (hospital department) and added, "We do not specifically provide coverage for hospice expenses."

A third New England group of two companies checked all services and by way of elucidation of Question 4, included a memorandum from their home office concerning hospices. Following are portions of that memo:

1. The described services to the patient would generally be covered under our Major Medical policies at the out-of-hospital coinsurance (most commonly 80 percent): but with so many of our policies containing family annual maximum expense out of pocket, by the time a person is ready for the services of a hospice, we'll most likely be paying 100%.
2. We write so little basic that does not also have a superimposed Major Medical, that there would appear little reason to consider the situation under basic alone. The mandated Home Health Care coverages in [state] and elsewhere would have a bearing on a basic (only) coverage.
3. Services to family members, if the charge may be isolated, would not be covered, except as treatment of his/her own illness—perhaps at 50% if the treatment is psychiatric.
4. Bereavement services could be covered only as in 3 above. Until there are more hospices (perhaps by then the word will have legislative definition), why don't we ask a hospice to approach us before the fact (when they are considering accepting the patient), convince us to agree to pay a specified amount as a means of loss control, and so convinced we could agree to pay.

Blues

An eastern Blue, in qualifying 3f (other), said, "Major medical coverage would provide benefits. However, no claims have been issued from a hospice to date." They further qualified with, "Services must be medically necessary and reasonable.'' An eastern Blue, explaining 3c (home care) wrote, ''Medicare home health benefits regulations.'' An eastern Blue fleet of 72 companies that checked 3c (home care) indicated that the home health services are provided currently under Medicare but that Blue Cross will provide home health benefits in the future and that some plans currently have hospice benefits. A western Blue that checked 3a (separate facility) and b (hospital department) explained, ''We recognize hospice services as being a skilled nursing facility type of benefit and level of care.''

A midwestern Blue checked 3b (hospital department) and d (multidisciplinary team) and qualified, ''To the extent of the various subscriber policies available in our area, such as limited to 120, 365, or 720 days based upon the medical necessity for hospital services.'' Finally, an eastern Blue which indicated they provide no hospice services said that they were ''presently considering parameters for hospice benefits.''

Question 5

If you do not provide hospice benefits, are you considering providing in the future?

Only 17 (13 percent) of the total 129 net responses indicated that they are considering providing hospice benefits (see Table 9-8), but from Table 9-7 we can see that there are 107 companies that do not provide benefits. Therefore, the 17 ''yes'' answers above represent 17 percent of the 99 companies that do not provide hospice benefits (see Table 9-6). Since the ''yes'' and ''no'' answers above total 120 instead of the 107 from Table 9-7, we can conclude that 13 companies that provide hospice benefits erroneously answered this question. If we assume that all 13 answered ''no,'' and if we then reduce the 103 ''no''s to 90, the ''no'' responses would still represent 84 percent of those companies not providing hospice benefits. Therefore, the overwhelming majority of the companies that do not provide hospice benefits are not considering providing in the future.

A midwestern Blue which indicated it provided services 3b (hospital department) and d (multidisciplinary team) checked ''Yes'' to Question 5 and added the following statement: ''Considering providing coverage on a pilot basis in other than a hospital setting.''

Question 6

If no, and it could be demonstrated that hospice care would be less costly than acute general hospital care, would your company consider paying specific hospice benefits?

Table 9-8 If you do not provide hospice benefits, are you considering providing in the future?

	Independents	**Fleets**	**Blues**	**Total**
Yes	7	2	8	17
No	73	7	23	103
No response	3	1	5	9

Question 6 leads directly from Question 5. The sum of the "yes," "no," and "uncertain" answers to this question is 113. The total "no" answers to Question 5 is 103. Therefore, ten companies answered this question erroneously. Nevertheless, using the data in Table 9-9, we can make some general observations—if we keep in mind that this survey is not a statistically valid sampling of the practices of all insurance companies that write health and medical insurance.

Since 28 responded "yes" and 71 responded "uncertain," we might conclude that 99 (88 percent) of the 113 respondents would possibly consider paying specific hospice benefits. We might conclude that the overwhelming majority of the respondent companies are interested in learning if hospices are potentially cost-effective.

Question 7

If any of your companies are Medicare fiscal intermediaries, do they pay benefits for hospice services?

Table 9-9 If no, and it could be demonstrated that hospice care would be less costly than acute general hospital care, would your company consider paying specific hospice benefits?

	Independents	**Fleets**	**Blues**	**Total**
Yes	18	2	8	28
No	13	1	0	14
Uncertain	48	6	17	71
No response	4	1	11	16

Table 9-10 If any of your companies are Medicare fiscal intermediaries, do they pay benefits for hospice services?

	Independents	Fleets	Blues	Total
Yes	0	1	4	5
No	1	0	20	21
Uncertain	1	0	1	2
Other	0	0	2	2
No response	81	9	9	99

There were 36 "yes" responses to Question 2, Is your company or are any companies in the fleet a Medicare fiscal intermediary? This would mean that the "yes-no-uncertain-other" answers to Question 7 should total 36 also, but they total 30 instead. Therefore, six companies that are MFIs failed to respond to Question 7.

Note that only 5 of the 36 MFIs mentioned in Question 2 pay hospice benefits. Of these five, four are Blues. Yet the Blues from Question 2 total 33. Therefore, only 12 percent of the Blues that are MFIs pay hospice benefits. From some of the responses to Question 4, it appears that the benefits provided under Medicare would be primarily home health services and skilled nursing facility services.

Three Blues, all of which are MFIs, had additional comments to add:

- "Yes—if it is billed as a *covered* acute service."
- "No—not classified as a skilled nursing facility—if hospices were so classified, then benefits could be considered based upon the type of care received, i.e., supportive vs. skilled nursing care."
- "Uncertain—to the extent such services constitute hospital or SNF [Skilled Nursing Facility] level of care."

Question 8

Comments or suggestions.

The most expeditious manner to record the responses to this question is to quote the ideas most frequently expressed by the respondents.

Independent companies

"As our plans pay specifically while confined to legally constituted hospital the only way payment could be considered is under b of Question 3 [separate department of general hospital]."

"Our policies provide benefits for acute care. Most of our policies are of a supplemental nature."

"Interested in this concept—very new to me."

"Our current health products contemplate coverage for hospital charges and physician's services."

"None of our contracts would cover any service other than the treatment of any illness or injury."

"We would consider charges for any medical care the patient received while confined in a hospice, but other charges would not be eligible."

"Some hospitals have a program whereby their staff members, priests, pastors, doctors, etc., consult with such families. Expenses for such programs would probably be part of hidden daily room charges or physician charges."

"Before we could consider developing benefits for specialized services of this type, there would have to be a customer demand and a sound actuarial basis for determining cost and rates."

"Many of our policies will cover portions of hospices' treatment under existing plan provisions. One of the critical questions we're wrestling with is whether some or all the care is custodial in nature."

"The description in your letter is somewhat limited as to the actual care provided the patient. Our policies provide benefits only for the care and treatment of an illness or injury therefore, we would not be able to provide benefits for the supportive care of the family of a terminally ill person."

"The hospice concept for the terminally ill is good only if meaningful and positive services can be performed only in such a setting, as distinct from, e.g., the home."

"We haven't encountered any claims for confinements to a hospice. As a result we've given no consideration as to coverage for expense from such an institution."

"If the services of a hospice team (I don't know what you mean by a multidisciplinary team) were billed by a hospital, our major medical policy would probably provide benefits as a 'hospital service or supply.'"

Fleets

"We are not aware of the existence of hospice benefits nor of any carriers that provide such benefits. We would appreciate any information you might have to bring us up to date on that subject." (Fleet of six companies)

"There is little doubt that hospice services provided to the patient by a recognized general hospital and billed for by the hospital would be a covered expense under most plans, providing it does not lapse into custodial care. Custodial care is not a covered expense." (Fleet of seven companies)

Blues

"Blue Cross of the . . . area is supportive of hospices, provided the hospitals are willing to convert existing beds for this service. It is important that our position is not mis-interpreted by hospitals and other providers to mean new construction and expansion, since we would not be responsive to such undertaking by these facilities under the banner of 'a service to the community.'"

"Our plan recently undertook a study of hospices; A pilot program is under development."

"We are presently studying the possibility of including home health care hospice services provided by multidisciplinary health care professionals. Consideration is being given to hospice qualifications to include licensure as a home health care agency, endorsement by the local county medical society and the American Cancer Society. We anticipate that we will be offering these services as a benefit of some of our Blue Shield business contracts in the relatively near future."

"Our certificates do not have any provision to provide benefits for hospice services the family may receive in connection with preparation for and support before and after death."

"We are not actively considering covering care in a hospice at this time; however, we are informally researching the topic, and therefore we are eager to assist you in whatever way we can."

"Blue Cross of . . . provides benefits according to the level of care rendered. Benefits are not payable for services that could be rendered by less than a skilled person."

Finally, one of the independent companies included a consummate letter, the following cogent paragraphs of which are quoted with permission:

> If the service is provided by the hospital and is included on the hospital's bill along with other hospital services, it is likely that Farm Bureau Life's Major Medical Policy would provide some coverage. It is not included as a named and defined benefit under the policy, therefore, no rating factors were added for this benefit in calculating the premium for the policy. The lack of concrete benefit limits would, in fact, make it difficult to actuarially calculate a premium for this benefit.
>
> Your definition of hospice includes "palliative and supportive care for terminally ill patients and their families." It is unlikely any insurer would be willing to provide such coverage for the

> family of a patient because of the dubious need for such coverage and the obvious opportunities available for abuse of such coverage. In other words, it would be nearly impossible to eliminate antiselection with such a diverse group as a family.
>
> If it could be shown that total claim costs for a terminal patient could be reduced through hospice care, there is no doubt insurers would be interested in providing specific hospice care. There is no one more interested in reducing the high cost of health care than the insurance industry. This is especially true with the increasing possibility of government intrusion in this area.[19]

Summary and Conclusions

The response rate to the mailed questionnaire was 25 percent, about the expected average. Although 145 total responses were received, some of these responses were from insurance groups or fleets representing an unknown additional number of individual companies. About 200–300 total insurance companies may be represented.

Approximately 28 percent of the net responses indicated they are Medicare fiscal intermediaries. Thirty-three of the 36 Blues (92 percent) indicated they are MFIs.

Only 17 percent of the net responses provide hospice benefits. (Throughout this chapter reference has been made to some insurance companies' providing or not providing hospice benefits. This has been a shorthand method of indicating that the specific insurors are providing or not providing *some* hospice benefits. Generally, the only services for which hospices receive insurance reimbursement payment are all medical nursing health services in which there is a "laying on of the hands." Counseling and bereavement service benefits are almost nonexistent.) Fifteen companies provide benefits for services provided in a separate department of a general hospital, eight companies provide home care service benefits, and three provide benefits for services provided in a separate hospice facility. To date, only one free-standing hospice facility exists in the United States—Hillhaven Hospice in Tucson, Arizona. Under construction is Hospice, Inc., in New Haven, Connecticut. Soon to open will be Kaiser-Permanente Hospice in Los Angeles, California. From the questionnaire responses it appears that Blue Cross/Blue Shield of Arizona is paying Hillhaven Hospice benefits as a skilled nursing facility. The eastern fleet of two companies apparently will pay a hospice benefits as a separate facility when approached. Apparently, the independent midwestern insurance company that answered that it would pay benefits for services provided in a separate hospice facility considers a hospice and a hospital to be synonymous.

Apparently few, if any, policies provide hospice benefits as a defined policy benefit. Some benefits would be provided for services furnished by a hospice under some basic, major medical, or comprehensive plans, but most companies do not provide for custodial care of terminally ill patients. The Medicare benefits that are reimbursable usually include those medical nursing services in which there is a "laying on of the hands." This would include some, but not all, home health services and in-facility services.

Several companies indicated that they are involved in researching the hospice concept. At least one indicated it was engaged in a pilot project. Although only 13 percent of the net respondents indicated that they are considering providing hospice benefits in the future, 88 percent would possibly consider paying hospice benefits if hospices could be demonstrated to be cost-effective.

A number of respondents felt that their benefit practices would be influenced by licensing practices of the states. Some felt they should be licensed as separate, legally constituted hospitals; others, as skilled nursing facilities; still others, as newly to be defined facilities or parts of existing organizations; and a few, as home health agencies.

Since so few hospices are in operation, most insurance companies have not experienced claims for hospice benefits. The great bulk of companies were not sure what in actuality a hospice does for terminally ill patients. Many apparently cannot grasp the notion of the patient *and* the family as the unit of care. The pervading existing philosophy of payment for *cure*, but not for *care*, came through quite clearly in the comments and letters that were submitted. Numerous companies indicated that their policies provide benefits only for the care and treatment of an illness or injury.

The concept of supportive care for the family is much misunderstood. Craven and Wald state that the bereaved are more vulnerable to physical and psychological disease; care for the survivors, therefore, is as legitimate a concern of health professions as preventive medicine.[20] Sylvia Lack has written that, in the first year after bereavement, there is an increased vulnerability to illness reflected in a 40 percent increase in the mortality rate of widows.[21] Richard Lamerton has said that part of the care of the dying is care of the bereaved; they are two sides of the same coin.[22] The Royal Victoria Hospital's excellent *Palliative Care Service: October 1976 Report* indicated that both psychological and somatic decompensation occurs among the bereaved. Included in the list of recorded disabilities are psychophysiologic illnesses, psychoneurotic conditions, coronary artery disease, insomnia, anorexia, and alcoholism.[23] Because of these manifestations in the bereaved, it appears that recognition of preventive care in the early stages of anticipatory grief[24] could be less costly to society in the long run. Compare, if you will, the potential costs of psychological counseling for the family in the early stages of the patient's terminal illness with the costs of prolonged hospitalizations for mental and physical disorders that arise after the patient's death.

HCFA DEMONSTRATION PROJECTS

On October 5, 1978, HEW Secretary Joseph Califano announced at the National Hospice Organization annual meeting in Washington, D.C. that Health Care Financing Administration (HCFA) would be conducting demonstration projects with organizations providing hospice services. This announcement subsequently appeared in the *Federal Register*.[25] As indicated in the invitation to bid, the purpose is to solicit demonstration sites where hospice services will be provided to Medicare and Medicaid beneficiaries and paid for by the Medicare and Medicaid programs. Central to these demonstrations will be an independent evaluation to assist HEW in making policy decisions regarding coverage of hospice services.

According to the invitation to bid, "waivers of Medicare coverage and reimbursement requirements and exclusions will be granted to successful respondents to permit payment for hospice services to patients with a life expectancy of six months or less." Of significant importance is the fact that the federal government recognizes that reimbursement policies are inadequate for hospice patients. The invitation to bid included the following examples of Medicare requirements and exclusions for which waivers could be requested:

> Medicare waivers for *in-home* hospice services may include:
>
> a. Waiver of the "home-bound" requirement for home health services.
> b. Waiver of the exclusion of drugs and biologicals provided in the home. Palliative drugs medically recognized and accepted will be reimbursed by the Medicare program. HCFA will determine on an individual hospice basis whether coverage and reimbursement will extend to prescription drugs such as anti-emetics, anti-depressants, and steroids.
> c. Waiver of the "skilled nursing requirement" so that payment will be made for services which are considered a custodial level of care.
> d. Waiver of the requirement for a new plan of treatment upon a patient's discharge following re-institutionalization. Because

some hospice patients will be institutionalized to stabilize their conditions, the current Medicare requirement that a new plan of treatment be established at each discharge may be waived.

e. Waiver of the current limits of 100 home health visits allowed under Part A of Medicare. Coverage of in-home hospice services may be expanded under Part A of the Medicare home health benefit with no numerical limits.
f. Waivers of the Medicare provisions relating to a three-day prior hospital stay, establishment of a plan of treatment by a physician within 14 days of discharge from a hospital or skilled nursing facility (SNF) and treatment for a condition treated in the hospital or SNF.
g. Waiver of exclusion of reimbursement for bereavement counseling to the family by a nurse or other qualified professional after the death of a hospice patient.
h. Waiver of restrictions on reimbursement for visits by psychologists, psychiatrists, and other qualified professionals made to the hospice patient and family.
i. Waiver of restrictions on reimbursement for visits made by the hospice team to hospice patients who have been reinstitutionalized.
j. Waiver of applicable coinsurance and deductibles for hospice services which are approved during the demonstration.
k. Waiver of the current Medicare cost reimbursement principles for hospice services if respondent proposes and HCFA accepts an alternative reimbursement system (e.g., capitation, prospective rates, etc.).
l. Waiver of the requirement that a patient must be in need of skilled nursing care, physical therapy, or speech therapy in order to utilize home health benefits.

Medicare waivers for *inpatient* hospice services may include:

a. Waiver of current Medicare cost reimbursement principles for services provided by hospitals and SNFs if a respondent proposes and HCFA accepts an alternative reimbursement system.
b. Waiver of the level of care requirements which must be satisfied before a patient can receive covered hospital or SNF services.
c. Waivers of the Medicare requirements for a three-day prior hospital stay, transfer within 14 days of discharge from a

hospital, and treatment for a condition treated in the hospital.

d. Waiver of the current limits on hospital and SNF days, scope and duration of benefits such that limits on the stay in a hospital-hospice and SNF-hospice will not be applied.
e. Waiver of deductible and coinsurance for a patient admitted to an institutional hospice.
f. Waiver of the limitations of the "benefit period" for admission to and coverage of services provided by institutional hospices.

STANDARDS FOR A HOSPICE PROGRAM OF CARE

Finally, mention must be made of standards for a hospice program of care. Since reimbursement of health services by third-party payers is tied so closely to legislation and subsequent regulations, the National Hospice Organization (NHO) has a committee hard at work developing standards derived from the NHO definition of hospice (see Chapter 2).

Although the NHO definition of hospice is brief, the NHO Standards Committee's interpretation of the definition leads to guidelines and standards that will form the basis for hospice development and evaluation. These guidelines in turn will form the basis for an accreditation manual, which inspection teams will use in certification and ongoing evaluation of hospice programs and hospice care.

There are various types of programs that provide care for the dying and their families. However, the word *hospice* is now a nationally registered service mark, as determined by the U.S. Patent and Trade Mark Office on February 14, 1978. The service mark was awarded to Hospice, Inc. of New Haven, Connecticut, which will transfer ownership to the NHO.[26] Therefore, the NHO will be responsible for establishing guidelines and standards for licensed use of the name *hospice*. Unauthorized use of the service mark is prohibited. Consequently no program of care will be certified as hospice by the NHO unless that program meets all aspects of the accepted definition and complies with the standards and guidelines. The definition and its amplification serve to differentiate certified hospice programs from other programs of terminal care that differ qualitatively and quantitatively from hospice programs.

Since federal and state governments will be scrutinizing these NHO requirements in establishing their reimbursement policies for federal and state health programs, standards and certification are important to all hospices. As the survey of insurance companies documented, insurance companies establish their reimbursement policies based in part on the licensing category of the health provider as well as on reimbursement policies promulgated by the federal and state governments.

THE BLUE CROSS AND BLUE SHIELD POLICY

A statement regarding hospice care and payment for hospice services was approved November 8, 1978 by the boards of the Blue Cross and Blue Shield Associations. Because the Blues' experience with hospice care is limited, the statement is a preliminary position that will evolve into a more permanent policy as the development, cost, utilization, and quality of hospice services are studied and evaluated further.

Briefly, the Blues support the basic concepts and philosophy of hospice care. Based on the overall criteria of demonstrated community need, medically acceptable standards of quality, and efficient, economical delivery of hospice care, the following principles will be used to determine payment for hospice services:

- Initial payment for hospice services should be made on a pilot or demonstration basis with a limited number of providers.
- Payments for services should, where possible, be made under existing benefit provisions or modifications of existing benefit provisions.
- Patients must meet written, detailed definitions of benefit eligibility.
- Hospice services to be paid for must have specified purpose and scope.
- Hospice services should be medically necessary and appropriate and be provided over a reasonable duration of time.
- Incentives that encourage delivery and use of the most economical and efficient hospice services should be provided in benefit and payment terms.
- Payments for services of a hospice program of care generally should not exceed payments for a program of acute inpatient services that would be available and medically appropriate for the same patient.[27]

Readers wanting further information are referred to the entire statement. Appropriate Blue Cross or Blue Shield representatives can supply additional information.

The demonstration projects announced by Secretary Califano and the approach taken by the Blue Cross and Blue Shield Associations toward provision of hospice services are positive steps forward. The private insurers throughout the nation should study closely the policy of these associations and monitor closely the progress of the HCFA demonstration projects. They can then modify their own health and medical insurance policies to provide insurance services for changing societal needs.

NOTES

1. Martin S. Feldstein, "The Medical Economy," *Life and Death and Medicine: A Scientific American Book* (San Francisco: W. H. Freeman & Co., 1973), pp. 112–19.

2. Parker Rossman, *Hospice: Creating New Models of Care for the Terminally Ill* (New York: Association Press, 1977), p. 216.

3. Ibid., p. 149.

4. Ibid., p. 216.

5. Janet Plant, "Finding a Home for Hospice Care in the United States," *Hospitals* 51 (July 1, 1977): 53–62.

6. Sheilah Kast, "Hospice: A New Way to Combat the Loneliness of a Loved One's Final Days of Life," *Washington Star*, November 28, 1977.

7. Sylvia Lack, "I Want To Die While I'm Still Alive," *Death Education* 1, no. 2 (Summer 1977): 165–76.

8. Ibid.

9. "Hospice Care Covered," *Modern Healthcare* 8 (April 1978): 30.

10. William Lamers, in testimony at California Legislature, Assembly Committee on Health, Public Hearing on Hospices, Santa Barbara, California, December 1, 1977.

11. Rossman, p. 217.

12. Lack, loc. cit.

13. Feldstein, op. cit.

14. Francis B. Kelly, *1977–1978 Nationwide Hospital Insurance Billing Directory* (Los Angeles: Francis B. Kelly & Associates, 1977), p. 4.

15. Ibid.

16. Claire Selltiz, Lawrence Wrightsman, and Stuart Cook, *Research Methods in Social Relations*, 3rd ed. (New York: Holt, Rinehart and Winston, 1976), p. 297.

17. Kelly, passim.

18. According to Kelly (pp. 4–5), many insurance companies belong to what are called fleets or groups of insurance companies. In some instances, all companies in the fleet have all health claims paid by the same office(s). In other instances, the companies in the fleet have different claims offices. Generally, all companies in an insurance fleet will give assistance or information of claims for other companies in the fleet.

19. Letter from Harry J. Solliday, Product Research and Development Analyst, Farm Bureau Life Insurance Company, West Des Moines, Iowa, October 27, 1977.

20. Joan Craven and Florence Wald, "Hospice Care for Dying Patients," *American Journal of Nursing* 75 (October 1975): 1,816–22.

21. Sylvia Lack, "Philosophy and Organization of a Hospice Program," Unpublished paper, n.d.

22. Richard Lamerton, *Care of the Dying* (Westport, Conn.: Technomic Publishing Co., 1976), p. 124.

23. *Palliative Care Service: October 1976 Report* (Montreal: Royal Victoria Hospital, McGill University, 1976), p. 98.

24. Bernard Schoenberg et al., eds., *Anticipatory Grief* (New York: Columbia University Press, 1974).

25. HEW, "Medicare and Medicaid Hospice Projects," *Federal Register* 43, no. 209 (October 27, 1978): 50,376–8.

26. *Hospice in America* (New Haven: National Hospice Organization, [n.d.]), p. 11.
27. "Initial Statement on Hospice Care and Payment for Hospice Services," Approved November 8, 1978 by the Boards of the Blue Cross and Blue Shield Associations.

Chapter 10
Legislation

One of the greatest delusions in the world is the hope that the evils in this world are to be cured by legislation.

Thomas B. Reed,
in a speech in the House of Representatives, 1886

The imbricative issues surrounding the hospice concept, for example, the definition of death, euthanasia, the right to die, and suicide, have been debated by physicians, attorneys, legislators, philosophers, and theologians for many years. The debate continues. Some states have taken legislative action in certain of these areas, but, because of the emotion surrounding these problems, both the oral and written public debates will continue to be heard, until, slowly, one by one, each of the states enacts legislation that will protect all its citizens in this important arena of human rights.

RIGHT-TO-DIE LEGISLATION

On September 30, 1976 California became the first state to enact legislation* prescribing a procedure whereby people may provide in advance for the withholding or withdrawing of medical care in the event they should suffer terminal conditions brought about by illness, disease, or injury. The person must formally execute a directive in the form and manner prescribed by law. If all the requirements are met, the act relieves physicians, licensed health care professionals, and health care facilities from civil liability, criminal prosecution, or charges of unprofessional conduct for withholding or withdrawing life-sustaining procedures pursuant to the directive.

The directive must be signed in the presence of two witnesses; if the patient is in a skilled nursing facility, one of the witnesses must be a patient advocate or ombudsman designated by the State Department of Aging. The witnesses cannot be related to the declarant by either blood or

*The Natural Death Act (AB 3060, Keene), which became effective January 1, 1977.

marriage and may not be entitled to any portion of the declarant's estate under will or by operation of law. Furthermore, neither the attending physician nor any employee of the physician or the health care facility can serve as a witness. The current act imposes heavy burdens on the attending physician, who is responsible for assuring that the patient is mentally competent and for ensuring that the directive is legally executed and witnessed, in accordance with the patient's true wishes. (See Appendix E for guidelines and directive for the California Natural Death Act and Appendix F for a copy of the act.)

The California Natural Death Act (CNDA) is a first step that needs broader application. As a result of legislators' attempts to delineate all possible conditions and circumstances in which the law might have become applicable and to meet objections of critics, AB 3060 became encumbered with the restrictions and limitations of nine separate amendments.

The amendments came about because of strong objections from "pro-life" groups such as the California Pro-Life Council, a loose-knit but dedicated, religiously oriented group with roots in the antiabortion movement.[1] Its members picketed the capitol and packed hearing rooms, calling the bill a first step toward euthanasia and likening withholding or withdrawing of medical care to medical practices in Nazi Germany.[2] Other critics argued that the law would be used by doctors who have outright contempt for patients of certain ethnic or economic backgrounds.

Deficiencies of the California Natural Death Act

At this writing, the law has been in effect for approximately one and a half years. According to its proponents, there are few problems with the law, and yet, according to its critics, the law did not go far enough in its intent.* Following is a list of the law's deficiencies, all of which need attention in future amendments.

- The principal drawback of the CNDA is that it does not make an advance declaration legally binding to protect the person who may later become a terminal patient.
- Physicians, generally, may not be willing to inform their patients of their terminal conditions. Even though the physician must consult with another physician, the patient's physician has that ultimate responsibility. His or her judgment alone determines whether death is

*For the statement of intent, see the preamble to the California Natural Death Act, AB 3060, S7186.

"imminent." There may be concern about the effect of an inaccurate diagnosis; this is probably a remote possibility, but not an impossibility.

- The provisions of the CNDA are not common knowledge to many physicians and most of the public; therefore, the CNDA is not being used as frequently as perhaps it should be. This is a problem of public education that should be addressed by the legislature and health care providers.
- There is no force of law to require the physician to follow the directive. It is left entirely to the physician to decide whether the circumstances justify effecting the directive if such a directive is executed prior to the onset of a terminal condition. Californians who properly execute directives have no absolute assurance that their wishes will ultimately be carried out.
- The directive is valid for only five years, whereupon the person may re-execute a directive after a diagnosis of a terminal condition. Taken together under the provisions of the "14-day rule," whereby a directive becomes valid after 14 days from the pronouncement of the terminal condition, the "five years rule" is not inconsistent, since a patient with a terminal condition would have a life expectancy well under five years.
- The 14-day rule makes the CNDA a "Lingering Death Act" (in the words of Arthur Bernstein, counsel, Kaiser Foundation Hospitals and Health Plan), "a law for people who are reasonably alert while suffering a lingering death."[3] Hence it is very narrow and restrictive.
- The onus is placed on the physician to determine the legality of the directive, including the mental competence of the patient and whether the witnesses fulfill all the requirements of the law. However, can the physician know for certain that the witness will not benefit from the patient's death because of a condition in the patient's will?
- The law makes no provisions for tragic newborns, children with terminal illnesses, or acute catastrophic illness or injury.
- If the patient is not physically able to sign the directive although mentally competent, as may be the case in some neurological diseases, there is no provision for a relative or legal guardian to sign.
- A directive may be revoked by any one of three methods: physical destruction, written revocation, or oral communication to the physician. The oral communication should be stricken from the law to ensure the patient's intent to revoke. The law now permits oral communication to a person other than the physician, who in turn must communicate to the physician. There are too many possibilities of

incomplete communication where the physician would not learn of the patient's wishes and might carry out the provisions of the directive, with tragic consequences.

- The requirement for witnessing of the declaration by a representative of the State Department of Aging (patient advocate or ombudsman) appears to be unduly burdensome. The intent of this provision seems to be to protect patients from abuses in nursing homes; however, there is no evidence that the law's provisions have corrected any alleged abuses or that they in any way added to the purport of the act.
- Prohibiting as witnesses those with whom the patient would come in contact, such as the physician, the physician's personnel, or health facility personnel seems onerous. By eliminating as legal witnesses relatives and those who would be named in the patient's will to receive a portion of the estate, not many choices may be left to numerous terminally ill patients who might want to execute a directive. This problem should be corrected.
- A provision for distribution of the directive was overlooked in the enactment of the CNDA. The required document is not readily available, either through the health department or some other state agency. The question arises whether the standard form is actually required. If an individual case doesn't fit the standard form, can another type of form be used? If so, would it be valid?
- If a woman becomes pregnant after executing the directive, the directive is then held invalid. This means that that woman may be subjected to inhuman, undignified treatment to keep her alive against her wishes. Tubes, needles, resuscitative equipment, and all sorts of technology may be used to prolong her ultimate death from the terminal condition. Can this provision of the law be just?
- The directive refers to the point at which "my death is imminent." There is no definition of the word *imminent.*
- "Unprofessional conduct" and its consequences need to be defined.
- Although to some it may appear innocuous, issuing the directive is actually a complicated procedure. There should be no need to consult an attorney or to have the directive notarized (as may be required in subsequent legislation of other states). The patient's rights can be protected by requiring the second physician's consultation and declaration of terminality placed directly on the declaration together with that of the patient's physician.
- Under the present CNDA, different conclusions can be reached in very similar situations. Friedman relates the case of a renal dialysis patient at Stanford University Medical Center who asked to sign the directive. The hospital's legal counsel opined that the patient did not

fall under the law's definition of "terminal." Thus the patient's signing would not be binding on the physician unless the patient's condition was rediagnosed as terminal. A similar case at University of California Hospitals and Clinics involved a renal dialysis patient who suffered complications requiring 19 major surgical procedures. The patient signed a directive that was held to be binding on the physician. The patient wanted no more surgery, but without surgery there were no more body sites available for entry of the dialysis equipment. As a result of the directive, if the current body site becomes unusable, no new sites will be explored, ensuring quick death as a result of kidney failure.[4]

Alternatives to the California Natural Death Act

In January 1978 the National Conference of Christians and Jews, Inc. conducted a public conference entitled "Ways of Looking at Death: Bio-Ethics and Public Policy," a discussion of alternatives to the California Natural Death Act. There were 145 participants at the day-long UCLA workshop, including academic humanists, physicians, nurses, attorneys, religious professionals, social workers, hospital administrators, senior citizens, university students, teachers, and interested citizens. Following are two of the primary issues explored, with the participants' consensus responses.

Should one alternative to CNDA be promoting active euthanasia?

- Education is a prime responsibility. Death education should be part of the curriculum of public schools from early age through graduation to begin to aid future generations to understand and cope with the dying and death itself.
- Counseling—Death counseling should be available for dying individuals and their families.
- A "Terminal Care Review Committee" should be created that would take legal responsibility away from the attending physician in cases where withdrawal of life support systems decisions are made.
- Health care insurance should be revised to provide benefits for hospice care.
- Hospices should be considered as a viable, publicly supported alternative.

Do hospices/pain reduction centers provide a viable means of treating dying persons?

- The conference consensus to this question was affirmative. Furthermore, the conference supported this idea of public support for hospice/pain reduction centers for the dying. A further recommendation was a public policy change to support patients' deaths at home; provide laws to require insurance coverage of the cost of care for patients who choose to die in their own homes.[5]

The Society for the Right to Die has prepared a modification of the California Natural Death Act. This modification allegedly overcomes many of the objections to the CNDA. It is presented in Appendix G. The reader can contact the Society for the Right to Die directly with questions or for additional copies of the document. Their address is 250 West 57th Street, New York, New York 10019.

Other Right-To-Die Legislation

The deficiencies of the CNDA notwithstanding, it was, in September 1976, a unique and daring piece of legislation that became the model for seven other states that passed similar laws within the following nine months. The 8 states with right-to-die laws and the 27 states with right-to-die bills are listed in Table 10-1.

Table 10-2 compares the eight right-to-die laws in existence. They are all somewhat similar, but each one has one or more features that deviate from the California law. Of particular interest is the North Carolina law, which includes a definition of brain death.

Brain death is a term commonly used to describe a condition in which the brain is completely destroyed and in which cessation of function of all other organs is imminent and inevitable.[6] The complete and permanent absence of any brain-related, vital bodily function is recognized as death by Jewish, Roman Catholic, and Protestant scholars even if they may disagree among themselves on the precise theoretical foundations of this judgment.[7]

Without a brain, the body becomes the medium in which the energy-requiring states of organs run down and the organs decay. These residual activities do not confer an iota of humanity or personality. Thus, in the circumstance of brain death, neither a human being nor a person any longer exists.[8]

Living Will

CONCERN FOR DYING (formerly the Euthanasia Educational Council) has for years advocated that people so inclined should execute a document known as a living will. This document predates the natural

Table 10-1 Right-To-Die Legislation

State	Bill Number	Bill Date Enacted	Sponsor(s)
Alaska	H632	—	Miller & Rudd
Arkansas	H826 (Act 879)	March 1977	Wilkins
California	AB3060	Sept. 1976	Keene
Colorado	H1029	—	Howe et al.
Delaware	H2	—	Ridings
Florida	H8	—	Hazelton
Georgia	H1258	—	Rowland et al.
	H51	—	Wall et al.
	S322	—	Foster et al.
Hawaii	H445	—	Garcia & Yamada
	H36	—	Garcia et al.
	H485	—	Segawa et al.
	S353	—	Kawasaki et al.
Idaho	S1164	March 1977	Murphy
Illinois	H5	—	Epton
	H467	—	Ewell
Iowa	S81	—	Ramsey
	H2351	—	Clark et al.
Kansas	S297	—	Winter & Simpson
Kentucky	H195	—	Lindsay
Louisiana	H1085	—	Le Blanc
Massachusetts	H840	—	Nordberg
	S767	—	Mass. Medical Society et al.
Michigan	H5778	—	Hollister et al.
Minnesota	S84	—	Keefe et al.
Mississippi	H478	—	Miller
	S2125	—	Molpus
Missouri	H1019	—	Downing et al.
Nebraska	L400	—	Barnett
Nevada	A8	May 1977	Coulter et al.
New Jersey	A481	—	Froude
	A1071	—	Hurley et al.
	A1123	—	Weidel

Table 10-1 Right-To-Die Legislation (continued)

State	Bill		Sponsor(s)
	Number	Date Enacted	
New Mexico	S16	April 1977	Conway & Valentine
New York	A10321	—	Brewer & Hevesi
	S7932	—	Gold
	S4841	—	Leichter
	A2383	—	Hevesi et al.
	S2175	—	Lewis
North Carolina	S504	June 1977	Smith et al.
Ohio	H516	—	Stinziano
Oklahoma	H1334	—	Duckett
Oregon	S438	June 1977	Hallock et al.
Pennsylvania	S1110	—	Holl
Rhode Island	H5396	—	Daniel
South Carolina	S197	—	Rubin & Wise
	H2419	—	Harris et al.
Tennessee	H132	—	Scruggs
	S966	—	Nave
Texas	S148	June 1977	Farabee
Washington	H252	—	Adams et al.
	S2477	—	Gould et al.
Wisconsin	A1086	—	Medinger

Source: Reprinted by permission of the publisher from *Legislative Manual*, 1978 (New York: Society for the Right to Die, 1978), p. 6. © 1978 by the *Society for the Right to Die*, Inc., 250 West 57th Street, New York, New York 10019.

death acts, but, unlike the natural death acts, it is not legally binding; however, the assumption is that the caregivers will feel morally bound to abide by its provisions at the appropriate time.

Copies of the living will can be obtained by writing to CONCERN FOR DYING, 250 West 57th Street, New York, New York 10019. The living will is shown in Exhibit 10-1. Following is the prescribed method of using the living will:

1. Sign and date before two witnesses. (This is to insure that you signed of your own free will and not under any pressure from outside sources.)
2. If you have a doctor, give him a copy for your medical file and discuss it with him to make sure he is in agreement. Give copies to those most likely to be concerned if the time comes when you can no longer take part in decisions for your own future. Enter their names on the bottom line of the living will. Keep the original nearby, easily and readily available.
3. Above all, discuss your intentions with those closest to you, NOW.
4. It is a good idea to look over your living will once a year and redate it and initial the new date to make it clear that your wishes are unchanged.[9]

The living will is by no means a substitute for legislative mandates by each of the states. In those eight states that have right-to-die laws, people covered by the laws should consider executing the proper legal document and should not rely upon any previously executed living will. In those states with natural death acts, it is unlikely that the courts would look with favor upon a physician who might follow the mandate of a living will when the legal form could and should have been executed. Such a situation, although leading to the desired end result for the patient, could lead to tragic results for the physician.

On the other hand, in those 42 states without right-to-die legislation a living will might be interpreted in those states' courts as the express wishes of the patient within the confines of the circumstances of the case, and legal sanctions would probably not be taken. However, since such a will provides no guarantees, for preventive purposes, it is advisable for the citizens of those 42 states to press their legislators to enact some form of right-to-die legislation.

DEFINITIONS OF DEATH

Except for sudden, accidental death, death proceeds in distinct stages. Organs fail at different rates, and when the body begins to die, it does so from below upwards. Use of the legs is lost before use of the arms, the abdominal organs cease to function before those in the chest, and the feet are cold before the head.[10] Because all cells of the body do not die at the same time, physicians can no longer pinpoint death as occurring from four to five minutes after heart action and breathing have ceased.[11]

Table 10-2 Comparison of Right-To-Die Laws

State	Became law	Time after which directive must be reexecuted	Form provided	Hospital and physician legally protected unless negligent	Binding on physician	Can be executed by person in good health	In order to be binding, must be reexecuted after patient becomes terminal
California (A.B. 3060)	Jan. 1977	5 years	Yes	Yes	Yes, if directive signed 14 days after patient becomes terminal	Yes, but not binding unless patient is terminal	Yes
Oregon (S.B. 438)	June 1977	5 years	Yes	Yes	Same as California	Same as California	Yes
New Mexico (S.B. 16)	June 1977	None	No	Yes, but physician must show "reasonable care and judgment"	Yes, but no penalty if physician does not comply	Yes	No
Nevada (A.B. 8)	July 1977	None	Yes	Yes	No	Yes	No (but directive is not binding at any time)
Arkansas (Act 879)	July 1977	None	No	Yes	Same as New Mexico	Yes	No
North Carolina (S.B. 504)	July 1977	None	Yes	Physicians are protected; hospitals not specifically protected	No	Yes	Same as Nevada
Idaho (S.B. 1164)	July 1977	5 years	Yes	Yes	Same as New Mexico (if patient is terminal and cannot communi-cate)	Same as California	Yes
Texas (S.B. 148)	Aug. 1977	5 years	Yes	Yes	Same as California	Same as California	Yes

Source: Reprinted by permission of the publisher from Emily Friedman, "'Natural Death' Laws Cause Hospitals Few Problems," *Hospitals, Journal of the American Hospital Association*, 52 (May 16, 1978): 124–130, 148.

Void while patient is pregnant	Provides for an agent to act on behalf of a minor	Provides for "ombudsman" for a patient in a skilled nursing facility	Provision for revocation	Penalties for hiding, destroying, or falsifying directive or revocation	Other provisions
Yes	No	Yes	Yes	Yes	Physician must determine validity of directive and witnesses. Concealing evidence of revocation constitutes murder. Directive must be placed in patient's medical record.
No	No	Yes	Yes	Yes	Physician need not determine validity. Directive must be placed in patient's medical record.
No	Yes	No	Yes	Yes	Physician need not determine validity. Court must certify agent's decision when minor is involved. Minor may counter agent's decision. Directive must be placed in patient's medical record or physician's case file.
Yes	No	No	Yes	Yes	Physician need not determine validity. Directive must be placed in patient's medical record. Similar documents executed before law went into effect "have same effect" as directives executed under the law.
No	Yes	No	No	No	Physician need not determine validity. Physician need not certify illness as terminal except for minors and incompetent patients. Proxy may act for incompetent patient. Signer may request life-sustaining procedures.
No	No	No	Yes	No	Physician need not determine validity. Hospitals not specifically protected but can cite law as a defense. Clerk of court must validate directive. No age provisions. Brain death defined.
No	No	No	Yes	No	Physician need not determine validity. Only operative if patient is comatose or unable to communicate with physician. Specifically does not cover persons not signing directives.
Yes	No	No	Yes	Yes	Basically the same as the California law except (1) physician need not determine validity and (2) no provision for ombudsman for patients in skilled nursing facilities.

Now that world medicine has progressed into the organ-transplant era, the definition and determination of death, from both a medical and a legal point of view, has become an extremely urgent necessity. "The exact point of death is not so important as the certainty that the process has become irreversible," declared Charles L. Hudson of Cleveland, Ohio, the United States' chief delegate to the World Medical Association, at the association's August 1968 meeting.[12]

The pronouncement of death on the basis of irreversible cessation of all brain functions has become common. Nevertheless, this use of the concept of brain death has caused considerable controversy among physicians, lawyers, legislators, philosophers, and theologians.[13] In 1968, a distinguished panel of 13 physicians, lawyers, theologians, and philosophers drew up a recommendation that was later published in the *Journal of the American Medical Association*.[14] The report, commonly referred to as the Harvard Report, claimed that, "an organ, brain or other, that no longer functions and has no possibility of functioning again is for all practical purposes dead." The report suggested that pronouncement of death be based on a clearly irreversible coma. It recommended that patients could be judged dead on four grounds:

1. Total unresponsiveness to all stimuli, including extreme pain
2. No sign of reflexes, e.g., pupils of eyes not responsive to light
3. Person's inability to move or to begin to breathe on own
4. No sign of brain activity on an electroencephalogram (EEG)

The Harvard panel also recommended that the patient be retested at least 24 hours after being judged dead. This provision was added to cover those cases in which exposure to cold or the taking of a drug overdose may have been responsible for suppressed activity, rather than death. The report goes on to say that when the patient is hopelessly damaged, as defined above, the physician in charge, in consultation with one or more physicians who have been directly involved in the case, should declare death, and *then* the respirator may be turned off. These consultive physicians, however, should not be involved in any later effort to transplant organs or tissue from the deceased person. This is to avoid any appearance of self-interest by the physicians involved. Although the Harvard Report has no legal standing, the weight of the recommendations is morally binding on the medical community.

In a rather exhaustive 1976 report appearing in the *American Journal of Law and Medicine*, H.A.H. van Till[15] contends that the Harvard Report criteria for irreversible coma are not reliable for diagnosing death in comatose patients under resuscitation treatment. Van Till claims that the Harvard Report is seriously flawed and that the time has come for its rejection. He further claims that, "a patient diagnosed as dead under the Harvard criteria may be only apparently dead, but actually alive."[16]

> The Harvard Report, by using logically inconsistent reasoning, creates a very dangerous situation in which a comatose patient under resuscitation treatment might be declared dead and thereby left legally unprotected against a variety of surgical assaults—for example, organ removal, autopsy, or biomedical experiments—while the existence of some degree of perception, possibly including the perception of pain and the spoken word, is still a possibility; in other words, while the patient still might be alive, though incapable of showing it.[17]

Van Till presents the following arguments as a basis for rejecting the Harvard Report.

Contradictory Message. The Harvard Report argues that "The burden is great on patients who suffer permanent loss of intellect."[18] The Harvard Report then contends that such people may be considered dead. The contradiction seems obvious. To be burdened people must be alive. And if they are alive, it is illogical and impermissible to declare them dead.[19]

Inappropriate Arguments. The Harvard Report presents several pragmatic, rather than medical, reasons for physicians to declare patients dead: 1) to relieve the burden on patients' families, on hospitals and their staffs, and on those in need of hospital beds already occupied by comatose patients; 2) to facilitate organ procurement for transplantation; 3) to provide a greater degree of legal protection to those who intend to accomplish the foregoing.[20] Van Till contends that "to declare death to achieve practical ends is ethically and legally unacceptable."[21]

Lack of a Definition of Death. The Harvard Report does not define death itself. To suggest criteria for diagnosing death, without defining a target at which the diagnosis may aim, is to skip an essential step of the process.[22]

Illogical Reasoning Concerning Clinical Symptoms. The Harvard Report, by proposing that clinical symptoms of death that generally foretell imminent death in patients *not* under resuscitation treatment may be used to declare death in patients who *are* under resuscitation treatment,[23] is attempting to use analogous reasoning under essentially dissimilar circumstances. The fact that patients show no reactions (other than spinal reflexes) to stimuli does not prove that they do not feel the stimuli. They

Exhibit 10-1 A Living Will

TO MY FAMILY, MY PHYSICIAN, MY LAWYER, MY CLERGYMAN
TO ANY MEDICAL FACILITY IN WHOSE CARE I HAPPEN TO BE
TO ANY INDIVIDUAL WHO MAY BECOME RESPONSIBLE FOR MY HEALTH, WELFARE OR AFFAIRS

Death is as much a reality as birth, growth, maturity and old age—it is the one certainty of life. If the time comes when I, ______________________ can no longer take part in decisions for my own future, let this statement stand as an expression of my wishes, while I am still of sound mind.

If the situation should arise in which there is no reasonable expectation of my recovery from physical or mental disability, I request that I be allowed to die and not be kept alive by artificial means or "heroic measures". I do not fear death itself as much as the indignities of deterioration, dependence and hopeless pain. I, therefore, ask that medication be mercifully administered to me to alleviate suffering even though this may hasten the moment of death.

This request is made after careful consideration. I hope you who care for me will feel morally bound to follow its mandate. I recognize that this appears to place a heavy responsibility upon you, but it is with the intention of relieving you of such responsibility and of placing it upon myself in accordance with my strong convictions, that this statement is made.

Signed ______________________

Date ______________________

Witness ______________________

Witness ______________________

Copies of this request have been given to ______________________

____

____

____

Source: Reprinted with the permission of Concern for Dying, 250 West 57th Street, New York, New York 10019.

may simply be incapable of reacting to the stimuli in a manner recognizable to others.[24]

Patients Bear the Burden of Proof. Under the Harvard Report criteria, patients have the burden of showing that they are still alive by producing outwardly perceptible and recognizable signs of life. Otherwise, they will be presumed dead after a specific period of time.[25] It seems improper that patients should bear this burden of proof. Patients should be presumed alive until they are proved dead by the physician, without any unnecessary margin of doubt.[26]

Overrating of Electroencephalogram (EEG) Significance. The Harvard Report states that an isoelectric EEG reading is "of great confirmatory value" in diagnosing death.[27] The EEG is not reliable or decisive with regard to brain death.[28] At best, it may suggest that death (the cessation of all neuronal function in the brain) has occurred. It should not be used to confirm or to prove death.[29]

Equating of Brain Impairment with Brain Death. The Harvard Report establishes a standard for diagnosing a severe impairment of brain function that, after a specific time period, may be assumed to be irreversible, based upon statistical data.[30] But a major malfunction of the brain is not the same as a total loss of brain function. Uncertainty among scientists, including neurologists, makes it necessary that an irreversible loss of *all* brain function be shown before it is medically, ethically, and legally acceptable to declare death. The Harvard Report blurs the distinction between a *mal*functioning brain and a *non*functioning brain.[31]

Van Till further contends that to diagnose a comatose patient under resuscitation treatment as dead, it is enough to prove total and uninterrupted absence of oxygen (anoxia) in the brain for at least 15 minutes, except in the case of hypothermia, young age, and central nervous system depressants.[32] Finally, van Till claims that "negative readings from properly performed bilateral serial angiography of the intracranial carotid and vertebral arteries over a period of 15 consecutive minutes proves retrospectively that brain death has occurred, although the exact moment of death cannot be pinpointed."[33]

The significance of the Harvard Report and of van Till's critical disclaimer of most of its criteria is that the definition of death is still not as precise as we would expect that it be. For many years, the definition of death as given in *Black's Law Dictionary* (see glossary for definitions of death) was accepted by the courts, but since October 1977, 18 states have enacted a statutory definition of death.

Alaska	Michigan
California	Montana
Georgia	New Mexico
Idaho	North Carolina
Illinois	Oklahoma
Iowa	Oregon
Kansas	Tennessee
Louisiana	Virginia
Maryland	West Virginia

All of these 18 statutes recognize that death may be pronounced on the basis of irreversible cessation of brain function, but none describes in detail the specific criteria for determining brain death.[34] Each of the 18 statutes is one of three major types.

1. Laws providing alternative definitions of death—The major flaw of this type is the misconception that there are two types of death.[35]
2. The concept suggested by Capron and Kass, to remedy the defect of #1 and provide one definition that recognizes that death is a single phenomenon that can be determined by brain-related criteria only in situations where artificial support of respiratory and circulatory functions is being maintained.[36]
3. Follows suggestion of the American Bar Association, which recognized the need for a standardized statutory definition of death that minimized the risk of confusion from misunderstandings of semantics, medical technology, and legal sophistication, and that took into account recent developments in transplantation, supportive therapy, and resuscitation.[37]

The American Bar Association (ABA) conducted an extensive study of the definition of death. The ABA study committee surveyed 180 lawyers and 20 professionals holding both legal and medical degrees. From this study, the ABA's Committee on Medicine by the ABA's House of Dele-Definition of Death," which was approved by the ABA's House of Delegates on February 24, 1975. The definition, and the resolution of which it was a part, read as follows:

> Resolution
>
> WHEREAS, it is to the well-being of the public to cease all artificial life supports, respiratory and circulatory, after a human body is dead; and
>
> WHEREAS, it is currently medically established that irreversible cessation of brain function is determinative of death; and
>
> WHEREAS, in the current technology of organ transplants it is vital that the donor's gift be in the best cellular condition,
>
> THEREFORE, be it resolved: that the American Bar Association offers a *Current Definition of Death* as follows: For all legal purposes, a human body with irreversible cessation of brain function, according to usual and customary standards of medical practice, shall be considered dead.[38]

The American Medical Association took the tack that state medical associations were to urge their legislators to postpone enactment of definition-of-death statutes. The following statement was affirmed by the House of Delegates of the American Medical Association: "Death shall be determined by the clinical judgment of the physician using the necessary available and currently accepted criteria."[39]

LEGISLATION SURVEY

Background research for this work included a survey conducted to determine what legislation pertaining to hospices, terminally ill, euthanasia, and related topics exists or is pending at the state level in the United States and at the provincial level in Canada. This, of course, involves legislation covering death, definitions of death, right-to-die legislation, and the like. A secondary purpose was to identify those states and provinces most knowledgeable about and most receptive to the hospice concept.

There are relatively few hospices in the United States (or palliative care services, as they are known in Canada). In the early phases of the preliminary research, the question arose as to which states (and provinces) had made legislative provisions for hospice development, licensure, and reimbursement. Knowledge of the extent of such legislation could be useful in enabling the hospice industry to focus attention on those issues most critical to it.

If specific legislation could be identified and analyzed, such knowledge would be of great assistance in developing new hospice programs, determining the direction of emphasis for additional necessary legislation, and influencing state funding of hospice programs. Prior research revealed that such information had not been identified and gathered together in one source. Therefore, a need existed.

Methodology

Although personal or telephone interviews of representatives of the 50 states and 12 provinces would have yielded the most reliable information, a mail survey was decided upon as the most practical method of collecting the necessary information, despite the usually low response rate to mail surveys.

Because of the nature of this survey, and because of the limited number of correspondents (62), follow-up letters and, finally, telephone calls were used in an attempt to achieve a 100 percent response rate. Each letter (see Appendix H) was addressed to the director of health (or equivalent) of each of the 50 states and the 12 Canadian provinces. As a supplement to the main thrust of this survey, two additional letters of inquiry were mailed: one to the Canadian Department of National Health and Welfare and one to the United States Department of Health, Education, and Welfare. Both letters asked for information similar to that contained in Appendix H.

Results

A total of 62 requests for information was mailed; 60 responses were received, for a total response rate of 97 percent (see Table 10-3).

Generally, a 97 percent response rate to a mail survey would be considered remarkable, since a response rate of only 30 to 40 percent is usually expected.[40] However, because the mailing was so small, and follow-up letters and telephone calls were used, a 100 percent response rate was expected.

Because this survey did not lend itself to a statistical analysis, because the responses were desultory in some cases, and because not all answers were pertinent to the purposes of the survey, the balance of this section consists of quotations extracted from letters of those respondents with germane comments.

United States

Some correspondents mentioned that their states had either bills pending before the legislature or laws relating to the right to die, natural death act, living wills, or similar issues. However, since the replies were desultory, the research vehicle was inadequate to present a clear and true picture of right-to-die legislation. Table 10-1, presented earlier, gives a complete picture of right-to-die legislation as of the end of 1978.

Table 10-3 Summary of Responses to Legislation Survey

		Responses	
	Mailing	**Number**	**Percent**
States	50	49	98
Provinces	12	11	92
Total	62	60	97

Although the reply from the National Cancer Institute (NCI) of the Department of HEW did not directly address the issue of legislation, the following quotation has been selected as representative of the philosophical view of hospices held by a major health policy branch of the United States government. It thus sets the stage for the selected comments from the states.

> We should point out that hospice is not a hospital and not a nursing home. The hospice is inspired by a different philosophy of care, relates to different goals, and provides different services to an entirely different population of cancer patients. It would more than compromise and complicate the purpose and meaning of the program to have it initiated within a general hospital.[41]

Arizona. "We currently have an inpatient hospice licensed under our nursing care institution regulations [Hillhaven Hospice, Tucson] . . . . A visiting-nurse type of hospice will probably be licensed under our home health regulations . . . . An inpatient hospice may be more appropriately licensed as a special hospital."

California. "Assemblyman Gary Hart introduced AB 1586 in the 1977 legislative session, which would require the Department of Health to develop and evaluate at least two hospice pilot projects and report to the legislature effective hospice care techniques and what steps, if any, the state should take to encourage and facilitate such care. This bill will probably undergo several amendments before enactment expected in mid-1978. At this writing, a total of $160,000 is to be appropriated for the two-year study."

Connecticut. "Hospice [,Inc.] obtained a certificate of need as a Chronic Disease Hospital. Plans, et cetera (for construction of a facility), are revolving around that licensure code . . . . Euthanasia would fall under the felony statutes of murder or manslaughter, depending upon the mitigating circumstances."

Georgia. "House Bill 769 would authorize the governor to establish a Cancer Management Advisory Group to advise on issues such as the need for facilities for the terminally ill and related questions."

Indiana. "There is a growing interest in this program [hospice], which indicates, at some future date, legislative action may be drafted and/or enacted within this state."

Kansas. "At the present time, there are no state agencies or hospitals providing the services of a hospice other than the long-term care facilities which are, in a sense, skilled nursing-care facilities. The skilled nursing facilities provide most of the services which you have outlined."

Louisiana. "Louisiana's new definition of death . . . addresses itself primarily to the death of an individual's brain. This statute is embodied in Section III of Title 9 of the Louisiana Revised Statutes of 1950."

Maine. "The questions you ask are too broad to be answered in a short period of time. Indeed, your definition of a hospice includes most of the items on the entire continuum of care: acute, long-term, and maintenance, be it in the home or another institution."

Michigan. "The only legislation adopted in this state in this general area is that which defines death. [H4653, passed and signed June 1975.]"

Nevada. "The hospice concept is still in the talking stage . . . . Methods of funding or legislation have not been looked into."

New Hampshire. "At the present time, a program of hospice is in the talking stage . . . . Because any funding for this mechanism must wait until the next legislative session, it will probably not be pursued prior to 1979."

New Jersey. "There is presently a hospice in New Jersey [Riverside Hospice], which this department [Health] has been funding as a demonstration project . . . . There is currently no legislation pertaining to hospices . . . . As a result of the presence of Riverside Hospice, however, and in anticipation of possible similar programs, there have been recent discussions in the department about initiating specific regulations for such."

New Mexico. "Our health facilities licensure statute is found at Sec. 12-34-5, NMSA 1953. The term "health facility" is defined at Sec. 12-34-2 (E). The definition does not include 'hospice.'"

Oregon. "The state of Oregon has no organized program which compares with your "Hospice" definition. However, each hospital and long-term care institution provides "Hospice" services to those individuals and families needing such services. Additionally, the secular community provides such services."

South Dakota. "Those services provided under a hospice program, if inpatient, would fall under our SDCL 34-12 relating to hospitals and related institutions. There is nothing that prohibits these institutions from providing these services if they are an appropriately licensed and certified facility. Outpatient hospice services could also be available under provisions of SDCL 36-4, Physician Practice Act, 36-4A Physician's Assistant Act, or 36-9, the Nurse Practice Act. Conformance with these laws does not exclude the provisions of hospice service . . . . If a person aids in the death of another, he could be tried under the murder or manslaughter provisions of South Dakota's Criminal Code."

Virginia. "The definition of a medical care facility in the State's Certificate of Need Law would include a hospice should there be a movement to build such a facility in Virginia."

Washington. "This state's hospital licensing legislation and its rules and regulations are sufficiently flexible to accommodate licensure of a hospice service as a hospital . . . . The main deterrent appears to be third-party payment either through such organizations as the Blues or Medicare."

West Virginia. "There has been considerable interest by the Bureau of Public Health Nursing to increase home care of the terminally ill through visiting nurse associations and other nursing facilities."

Wisconsin. Attached to reply was Research Bulletin 76-4, *Definition of Death and Euthanasia,* prepared by Legislative Council Staff, revised December 31, 1976.

Wyoming. "In thirteen county public health nursing services certified as home health agencies, four county public health nursing services not certified and one hospital-based certified home health agency within this state home health services are provided to terminally ill patients. Through this service, professional nurses assist families in providing care for terminally ill patients on orders of private physicians. The nursing services are often provided on an intermittent basis through death at home or up to a day or so before death, when the patient goes to the hospital. The nurses help patients and families prepare for the loss of dying. After patients expire, the nurses generally continue to visit the families of those patients to give counseling through the mourning process."

Canada

The response from the Canadian National Department of Health and Welfare stated in part:

> In Canada, the provinces have jurisdictional authority in health matters; however, in situations where human life is the major issue of concern, these aspects are covered by the federal Crimi-

> nal Code. Reference in this instance is made to Sections 205 [Homicide], 206 [When Child Becomes Human Being—Killing Child], 207 [Death Which Might Have Been Prevented], 208 [Death From Treatment of Injury], 209 [Acceleration of Death], and 210 [Death Within Year and a Day] of the Criminal Code . . . . In addition, Section 14, on Consent to Death, is enclosed . . . . There is no known federal or provincial legislation, either actual or pending on the subject of euthanasia.
>
> The provinces have direct responsibility for the provision of health services to the well and unwell. The delivery of medical services and by extension the hospitals come under provincial jurisdiction.
>
> There is no known provincial legislation regarding hospices (as defined) or separate provisions pertaining to care of the terminally ill. In certain hospitals, however, there is a palliative and supportive care service in operation for the terminally ill. These services are functioning under the provincial health authority and receive payment for services under the provincial hospital and medical care programs . . . .[42]

Alberta. "The Dependent Adults Act of Alberta . . . provides for a mechanism for the appointment of a guardian of a dependent adult who can be empowered by the courts to make decisions respecting the health care of the dependent adult. It is conceivable that a guardian could be asked to make decisions respecting the health care of a dependent adult, which might relate to the termination of any treatment in the case of a terminally ill patient. It is, therefore, arguable that this legislation might empower the guardian to make decisions respecting euthanasia."

New Brunswick. "We have no palliative care units in any of our hospitals. The terminally ill patient may be accommodated in an active treatment hospital if intensive nursing care is required, but many terminally ill patients spend their last days in a nursing home. However, we are encouraging the family of the terminally ill to participate in the care with the aid of visiting nurses . . . and homemakers service under the auspices of the Canadian Red Cross."

Nova Scotia. "The English Common Law would provide the basis for establishing the duty of these various organizations [hospitals, nursing homes and homes for special care] toward the patient. I think that you will find generally in Canada that there is much less of a tendency to resort to legislative solutions in these matters than in the United States."

Ontario. "In Ontario, euthanasia is against the law. The practice of it would be considered murder . . . . Currently there are three pilot projects in long-term chronic care in the Province of Ontario . . . . They probably more aptly meet the needs of the terminally ill patient and are currently under ongoing evaluation as to the impact extension of long-term care would have on the delivery of Health Care services in the Province of Ontario."

Summary and Conclusions

The most significant survey finding was that not one of the respondents had any legislation in existence relating directly to hospices. Only one state, California, had a bill pending before the legislature. The California bill would require the establishment of at least two pilot hospice projects featuring Medi-Cal (Medicaid) reimbursement. By January 1, 1981, the conclusions and recommendations resulting from the pilot programs are to be reported to the legislature.

Incidentally, on December 1, 1977, the California Assembly Health Committee conducted an all-day hearing in Santa Barbara on the subject of hospices. The purpose of the session was primarily educational—both for members of the health committee and for the public—with hospice practitioners from all over the state presenting testimony on their experiences, the needs of developing hospices, and the need for future legislative aid. As Sidney Smith, executive director of Hospice of Santa Barbara, proclaimed at the hearing, "The Assembly Health Committee is to be commended for conducting the first legislative forum in the nation on the topic of hospices." However, Smith was apparently unaware that in the spring of 1977 the state of Connecticut had a significant hospice bill submitted to its legislature. The bill, signed into law in 1978, allows for the provision and reimbursement of home health services, including medical social services, for the terminally ill.

In a personal letter, Senator Hugh T. Farley of New York requested a copy of California AB1586. As Senator Farley indicated, "the New York State Coalition of Hospices is interested in establishing such an institution in New York State. It would [be] a help to receive a copy of your proposed legislation in order to aid us in writing a similar bill."[43]

Thirty-five states had one or more right-to-die bills pending before their legislatures at the end of 1977.[44] Additionally, eight states had right-to-die laws enacted in 1976 or 1977.[45] Of the 35 states with right-to-die bills before their legislatures in 1977, only 11 respondents mentioned that fact in their letters of response. The state that did not respond had one bill pending. Twenty-two respondents either indicated that they had no bills regarding terminally ill, euthanasia, or related topics or did not mention any such bills, responding instead with comments or information on other topics. There was no similar pending legislation reported in Canada.

Of the eight states with right-to-die laws, only three respondents mentioned that fact in their responses. Five respondents either indicated that they had no laws regarding terminally ill, euthanasia, or related topics or did not mention any such laws in the response.

Three respondents referred to an existing hospice operation in their respective states. Five indicated that there was interest in the hospice movement. Five states referred to licensing and certificate of need considerations. Two indicated that skilled nursing homes provide the services of hospices. One state has a bill pending that would authorize the governor to establish an advisory group to advise on issues related to the terminally ill, including the need for facilities. Two states indicated that they had legislation that defines death. Two states indicated that the practice of euthanasia would fall under their criminal codes; any person engaging in the practice would be subject to charges of murder or manslaughter. One respondent mentioned the issue of reimbursement as a probable deterrent to hospice development. Two states ıeferred to increased interest in home care for the terminally ill. As of early 1978, no state or province had any legislation covering the topic of hospices, and only one state, California, had a bill to study hospices pending before its legislature.

Subsequent Developments

In April 1978, subsequent to the survey, Congressman Douglas Walgren of Pennsylvania introduced a bill (HR 12358) in the House of Representatives that would provide for the development of standards for provision of hospice care and also provide for studies and demonstration projects in the provision of hospice care. By March 1, 1981, a preliminary report, and by December 1, 1981, a final report would be submitted to Congress. The bill was referred to the Subcommittee on Health and Environment on April 26, 1978; no action has been taken as of this writing. It appears that this bill will undoubtedly be amended or replaced by one or more bills, but some similar bill or bills will probably be enacted by Congress after 1979.

On the national scene, HEW has engaged a task force headed by Peter Libassi, HEW chief legal counsel, to prepare a report on hospices. This report is due to Secretary Joseph Califano by August 1, 1978. This report will undoubtedly form the basis for additional congressional activity.

In the summer of 1978, the state of New York passed legislation (S.9725 B) to establish a pilot program for hospices. The intent is to evaluate the use of hospices and aid in eventual certification and operation of hospices as part of the total health care system in the state. The pilot program includes three hospice models. Each model will follow up with a program of home care with backup patient beds in a) a special, autonomous unit of an acute-care facility or a nursing home; b) in a free-standing hospice facility; and c) whatever unit of a general hospital the patient may be admitted to. The program will begin prior to January 1, 1980 and will expire on March 1, 1983; the commissioner of health's findings and recommendations for legislation are to be reported on or prior to March 1, 1983.

On September 29, 1978, California Governor Edmund G. Brown, Jr. signed AB 1586 into law. As amended, it provides that the State Department of Health Services shall conduct at least two hospice pilot projects to establish regulations and levels of reimbursement for Medi-Cal (Medicaid) recipients and to evaluate hospice care. The pilot projects will be conducted for a period of one year beginning on or before April 1, 1979 and ending no later than April 1, 1980. A report is to be made to that legislature by April 1, 1980; conclusions and recommendations are to include at least the following issues:

1. An assessment of whether Medi-Cal reimbursement should be made available for hospice care; if so, recommendations on rates and regulations
2. An assessment of the quality and cost effectiveness of:
   a. Use of layperson volunteers for hospice care
   b. Hospital vs. traditional care
   c. Institutional vs. in-home hospice care
3. An assessment of the current and projected demand for hospice care in either newly constructed hospice facilities or in existing facilities

A sum of $160,000 was appropriated for the purposes of this act.

NOTES

1. "Right-To-Die Law Runs into Problems," *Los Angeles Times*, November 25, 1977, part II, p. 9.
2. Ibid.
3. Emily Friedman citing Arthur Bernstein, "'Natural Death' Laws Cause Hospitals Few Problems," *Hospitals* 52 (May 16, 1978): 124 ff.
4. Emily Friedman, "California Hospitals Design Natural Death Act Procedures," *Hospitals* 51 (November 16, 1977): 62–5.

5. "Ways of Looking at Death: Bio-Ethics and Public Policy II," Conference sponsored by National Conference of Christians and Jews, Inc., University of California at Los Angeles, January 17, 1978.

6. Frank Veith et al., "Brain Death: I. A Status Report of Medical and Ethical Considerations," *JAMA* 238 (October 10, 1977): 1,651–5.

7. Ibid.

8. Ibid.

9. CONCERN FOR DYING, 250 West 57th Street, New York, New York 10019.

10. Richard Lamerton, *Care of the Dying* (Westport, Connecticut: Technomic Publishing Co., 1976), p. 141.

11. E. Kenneth Froslid, "A Definition of Death," *World Book Year Book,* 1969, p. 407.

12. Ibid., citing Hudson.

13. Veith et al., "Brain Death: I," loc. cit.

14. "A Definition of Irreversible Coma: Report of the Ad Hoc Committee of the Harvard Medical School to Examine the Definition of Brain Death," *JAMA* 205 (August 5, 1968): 337–40.

15. H.A.H. van Till, "Diagnosis of Death in Comatose Patients under Resuscitative Treatment: A Critical Review of the Harvard Report," *American Journal of Law and Medicine* 2 (Summer 1976): 1–40.

16. Ibid.

17. Ibid.

18. Harvard Report, loc. cit.

19. van Till, loc. cit.

20. Harvard Report, loc. cit.

21. van Till, loc. cit.

22. Ibid.

23. Harvard Report, loc. cit.

24. van Till, loc. cit.

25. Harvard Report, loc. cit.

26. van Till, loc. cit.

27. Harvard Report, loc. cit.

28. van Till, loc. cit.

29. Ibid.

30. Harvard Report, loc. cit.

31. van Till, loc. cit.

32. Ibid.

33. Ibid.

34. Frank Veith et al., "Brain Death: II. A Status Report of Legal Considerations," *JAMA* 238 (October 17, 1977): 1744–8.

35. Ibid.

36. A. M. Capron and L. R. Kass, "A Statutory Definition of the Standards for Determining Human Death: An Appraisal and a Proposal," *University of Pennsylvania Law Review* 121 (1972): 87–118.

37. Veith et al., "Brain Death: II," loc. cit.

38. American Bar Association, *Report of the Committee on Medicine and Law*, 11, forum 300 (1976): 311.

39. "Definition of Death," *JAMA* 227 (February 18, 1974): 728.

40. George R. Allen, *The Graduate Students' Guide to Theses and Dissertations: A Practical Manual for Writing and Research* (San Francisco: Jossey-Bass, 1973), p. 56.

41. Letter from Lawrence Burke, Program Director for Rehabilitation Treatment, Rehabilitation and Continuing Care Branch, DCCR, NCI, December 15, 1977.

42. Letter from Robert H. Lennox, Senior Consultant, Child and Adult Health, Health Consultants, Canada Health and Welfare, Health Programs Branch, November 1, 1977.

43. Letter from Hugh T. Farley, Senator, State of New York, December 9, 1977.

44. *Legislative Manual, 1977* (New York: Society for the Right to Die, 1977), p. 6.

45. Ibid., pp. 3–6.

Chapter 11

U.S. and Canadian Hospices

I was hungered, and ye gave me meat:
I was thirsty, and ye gave me drink;
I was a stranger, and ye took me in.
Matthew 25:35

In addition to the reimbursement and legislative surveys presented in Chapters 9 and 10, a third survey was conducted to identify hospice programs, both existing and forming, in the United States and Canada. The intent was to compile a listing of each of the hospices and outline their salient organizational, operational, and demographic features. Such a compilation would be of interest and assistance to all other existing hospices and those in the planning stages. It could also become a resource for other organizations and individuals interested in developing hospice references.

Because there are relatively few hospices in the United States and few palliative care services in Canada, identification of those existing and developing programs was difficult. A specific hospice program was generally known only locally, usually to a relatively small population that might be associated in some way with the program. For instance, a person in Southern California generally would have no knowledge of a hospice program developing in a rural area of Minnesota, and an existing program participant in New York City probably would have no knowledge of a planned program in Phoenix. With few exceptions, most programs are being developed or have developed independently of other programs, with only people and organizations within a small geographical area involved in the development of the program.

METHODOLOGY

A two-page questionnaire and a letter of transmittal were designed (see Appendices I and J) and mailed to 149 organizations throughout Canada and the United States that were possible hospices or developing hospices. The questionnaire contained questions pertaining to ownership, programs and services, visitors, the unit of care, demographics, home care and inpatients, volunteers and personnel, diagnosis distribution, patient age distribution, reimbursement and funding, and overnight accommodations for families. The final question was a write-in for additional comments.

RESULTS

A total of 149 questionnaires were mailed. Seventy-one responses were received, for a response rate of 48 percent (see Table 11-1).

Active Hospices

There are more than the 57 active, planned, and community support group hospices shown in Table 11-1 in the United States and Canada. Only those that replied to the questionnaire are reported here. A short description of each of the 33 respondents follows. The information was current as of January 1978. Because most of the hospices mentioned below are in a constant state of development, current information may differ to some extent. Although some of the following organizations do not consider themselves to be true hospices, they do operate as such in many respects and are thus included and identified as hospices. The reader who would like more specific information about any hospice program in particular should contact that hospice directly. See Appendix A for names and addresses of hospice programs.

Bellin Hospice, Green Bay, Wisconsin. A 10-bed unit of Bellin Memorial Hospital (a nonprofit community hospital) provides inpatient palliative care, home palliative care, consulting and referral services, bereavement follow-up services, teaching, homemaker, spiritual, and social services. In operation since July 1977. Visiting times are seven days per week, 24 hours per day, with no age restrictions for visitors. The patient and the family are the unit of care. The population served is up to 500,000 and 95 percent of the patients come from up to 30 miles away. They provide home care services as a certified home health agency 24 hours a day, 7

Table 11-1 Summary of Responses to Hospice Survey

	Number	Percent
Active hospices	33	47
Planned hospices	23	32
Community support group	1	1
Not a hospice	14	20
Total	71	100

days per week and serve about 40 to 50 patients at any one time. The average daily inpatient census is five; the mean length of stay is 11 days. They have 18 volunteers in the program; each volunteer averages 12 hours per month after undergoing a 20-hour orientation. Full-time equivalent personnel: RN, 5.6; LPN, 7.0; social worker, 0.4; physician, 1.0; clergy, 0.5; administrative, 0.1. The patient's own family physician and pastor are actively involved in care of the patient. Admitting diagnoses are: cancer, 90 percent; kidney, 2 percent; heart and lung disease, 4 percent; progressive neuromuscular disease, 4 percent. Half of the patients are between 18 and 64 years of age, and half are 65 and over. For third-party reimbursement, Bellin is classified as an acute hospital. The revenue breakdown is: Medicare, 50 percent; Medicaid, 5 percent; commercial insurance, 30 percent; self-pay, 5 percent; philanthropy, 10 percent. Philanthropic funding comes from the church, memorials, and individuals. Although beds are not provided, patients' families are allowed to stay overnight either in the lounge or on chairs in patients' rooms.

Bethesda Lutheran Hospice, St. Paul, Minnesota. A 12-bed unit presently housed in the oncology unit of the nonprofit Bethesda Lutheran Hospital has provided inpatient palliative care, home palliative care, consulting and referral services, bereavement follow-up services, teaching, dietary, pharmacy, physical therapy, occupational therapy, homemaker, and spiritual services since July 1977. Normal visiting times are Monday through Friday, 7:30 A.M. to 4:00 P.M., with no age restrictions for visitors. The unit of care is the patient and family, with the family including "significant others." The population served is between 500,000 and 1 million, with 100 percent coming from up to 30 miles away. Home care can be provided to an unlimited number 24 hours per day, seven days per week. Average daily inpatient census is six; the average length of stay is 21 days. They have no volunteers at present but are recruiting. Full-time equivalent personnel: RN, 1.0; physician, 0.20; clergy, 0.33; administrative, 0.5. All the patients are admitted with cancer diagnoses, and 90 percent of the patients are between 18 and 64 years of age, with 10 percent being 65 years or older. Their entire funding comes from foundations. They have limited facilities for overnight stays of patients' families; a twin-size convertible bed and rollaways are available.

Boulder Hospice, Inc., Boulder, Colorado. A nonprofit corporation organized in June 1977 offers home care to 15 patients on a less-than-24-hour basis, consulting and referral services, bereavement follow-up services, teaching, and public education. The unit of care is the patient and family, and they offer bereavement services for the nonhospice population. They serve a population of 100,000 to 500,000, with 95 percent of the patients being at a distance up to 30 miles away and 5 percent at a distance of between 30 and 50 miles. They have 25 volunteers in the program who serve two to three hours per week after a 2½-day intensive training program and ongoing monthly inservice training. They have two clerical personnel funded by a Public Service Employment grant, and all other services are provided by volunteers including the executive director, the medical director, and all nursing personnel. All the patients currently are diagnosed with cancer. Funding comes from federal grants, church donations, and local individuals. Volunteers have donated space in their homes for families' overnight accommodations.

David M. Brotman Hospital, Culver City, California. This is a 38-bed oncology unit of the 550-bed investor-owned hospital. It provides consulting and referral services, bereavement follow-up services, teaching, social services, professional and paraprofessional counseling, and spiritual services. Visitors of all ages are permitted 24 hours per day, seven days per week. The unit of care can be either the patient, the family, or the patient and family. The unit serves a population base of greater than 1 million, with 70 percent coming as far as 30 miles, 20 percent up to 50 miles, and 10 percent between 50 and 100 miles. The average daily census is 30. They have 40 volunteers who each provide about six hours' service per week; volunteers meet weekly and get individual training supervision. Full-time equivalent personnel: RN, 5; LVN, 3; social worker, 1; physician, 8; administrative, 3; thanatologist, 1; clergy varies. Ninety percent of the patients are admitted with cancer diagnoses, 10 percent with blood disorders. Forty percent of the patients are between 18 and 64 years, and 60 percent are 65 years and older. The beds are classified as acute hospital for third-party reimbursement purposes. Revenue comes 30 percent from Medicare, 30 percent from Medicaid, and 40 percent from commercial insurance. No overnight accommodations are provided for families of patients.

Calvary Hospital, Bronx, New York. Under the control of the Archdiocese of New York as a nonprofit corporation, this 200-bed hospital provides inpatient palliative care, consulting and referral services, bereavement follow-up services, teaching, social services, recreation therapy, and spiritual services. The program was begun in 1900. They have no age restrictions for visitors, and visiting is allowed seven days per week, eight hours per day. The patient and family is the unit of care. All the patients from the greater New York City metropolitan area come from within a 30-mile radius. The average length of stay is 66.7 days. The average daily census is 105. They are planning home care services for the future. A total of 80 volunteers provide an average of 130 hours' service each per year. Full-time equivalent personnel: RN, 34; LPN, 11; social worker, 4; physician, 5; clergy, 3; administrative, 2; housekeeping, 18. All the patients are cancer patients; 40 percent are between 18 and 64 years, and 60 percent 65 and older. They are classified as a specialty hospital for third-party reimbursement. Total revenue by payer: Medicare, 36 percent, Medicaid, 54 percent, commercial insurance, 10 percent. Some funding comes from foundations, state government, and the church. They provide overnight accommodations for family members.

Church Hospital Corporation, Baltimore, Maryland. This is a 14-bed unit in an acute hospital, which is a nonprofit corporation. They provide inpatient palliative care, home palliative care, consulting and referral services, bereavement follow-up services, teaching, social services, homemaker, spiritual, physical therapy, and speech therapy. The program began October 1975. There are no age restrictions for visitors and visiting is permitted seven days per week, 24 hours per day. The unit of care is the patient. They serve 500 patients through the home care service on a seven-day-per-week, 24-hours-per-day basis. There are ten volunteers in the program who get an orientation and ongoing training. Full-time equivalent personnel: RN, 2; LPN, 3; social worker, 0.50; physician, 0.50; clergy, 2; administrative, 1; physical therapist, 0.75; speech therapist, 0.25. All the patients are admitted with cancer diagnoses, 10 percent under 18 years of age, 20 percent between 18 and 64 years, and 70 percent 65 years and older. All the funding is provided by hospital revenues: Medicare, 30 percent; Medicaid, 20 percent; commercial insurance, 20 percent; self-pay, 20 percent; other, 10 percent. No overnight accommodations are provided for patients' families.

El Camino Hospital, Mountain View, California. This public-owned hospital began its hospice program on February 15, 1978, through its Human Energy and Resources Team. They provide home care services, with inpatient palliative care provided as needed in various units of the hospital. Additional services provided are consulting and referral, bereavement follow-up, counseling, spiritual, and social services. There are no visitor age restrictions, and visiting is permitted seven days per week, 24 hours per day. The unit of care is the patient, the family, and the caregivers. Ninety-five percent of patients come from within 30 miles' distance, and 5 percent are from 100 or more miles. The home care services are provided 24 hours per day, seven days per week. Fifteen volunteers provide four hours per week service after a six-week intensive training course. The hospital staff—human support, nursing, social worker, chaplain—all work in the hospice program on a volunteer basis. All funding is provided from county funds. They do not as yet provide overnight accommodations for patients' families.

Haven of Northern Virginia, Inc. An all-volunteer nonprofit corporation, it provides services at no charge. The nurses provide supportive care, not primary care, often working as an extension of the public health and/or visiting nurses. Many of the referrals come from hospitals, nursing homes, and other health care agencies as well as physicians and nurses. In addition to nursing supportive care, other services offered are consulting and referral, bereavement follow-up, counseling, home helpers, spiritual, teaching, widows' and parents' groups, groups for teens, and social services. The program began September 1976. The unit of care is multiple, consisting of patient, family, patient and family, and extended family. All patients come from within a 30-mile radius and a population base of 500,000 to 1 million. The home care services are assigned to available professional volunteers, who serve up to 8 or 9 hours per day. Up to 250 patients can be served by 155 lay volunteers, who initially receive 30 hours of orientation followed by intensive inservice and advanced courses. Each lay volunteer provides 8 hours' service per week. Long-range care has been given to almost 250 families, short-range to another 300. Patients are admitted for the following conditions: cancer (67 percent); heart disease (4 percent); and accident, stroke, suicidal tendencies, and grief (29 percent). Four percent of the patients are under 18 years, 65 percent are between 18 and 64, and 31 percent are 65 and over. Funding comes from the church, individual donations, and private grants.

Hillhaven Hospice, Tucson, Arizona. A 39-bed, free-standing hospice unit (the first in the United States), it is a nonprofit subsidiary of Hillhaven Foundation. It provides inpatient and home care palliative services, consulting and referral services, bereavement follow-up services, teaching, homemaker, spiritual, and social services. The first patient was admitted in April 1977. There are no age restrictions for visitors, who have seven-days-per-week, 24-hours-per-day visiting privileges. The unit of care is the patient and family. The population served is up to 500,000, with 90 percent of the patients coming from up to 30 miles, 5 percent from up to 50 miles, and 5 percent from 100 miles or farther. Home care is provided seven days per week, 24 hours per day. The average daily inpatient census is 25. Average length of stay is 24 days. The 43 volunteers provide four hours per week of service after 8 hours' orientation, plus ongoing educational training. All the patients are admitted with cancer diagnoses; 60 percent are between 18 and 64 years of age, and 40 percent are 65 years or older. The beds are classified as skilled nursing facility beds for third-party reimbursement purposes. Funding is provided by a National Cancer Institute grant, Medicare, the county, commercial insurance, and private-pay patients. Two rooms in the facility are provided for overnight accommodation of patients' families.

Home Hospice of Sonoma County, Santa Rosa, California. This was, at the time of the survey, an unincorporated group in the process of becoming incorporated. They provide home palliative service 24 hours per day, seven days per week, consulting and referral services, bereavement follow-up services, teaching, spiritual, and community services referral. Their program began in July 1977. They serve a population base of up to 500,000, with all the patients coming from within a 30-mile radius and serve 20 or more home care patients. They have 50 volunteers who each undergo a one-semester hospice course at Santa Rosa Junior College. All of the patients have diagnoses of cancer; 30 percent are between the ages of 18 and 64, and 70 percent are 65 or older. All personnel are unpaid volunteers. The funding comes from foundation grants, donations, and hospice memberships. The hospice is primarily a counseling, referral, consulting, and support team, with medical and nursing responsibility that of the patient's physician and the Visiting Nurse Association.

Hospice Atlanta, Inc., Atlanta, Georgia. This is an essentially volunteer organization with both home care and day care. They plan no inpatient facility. Current activities are primarily educational. It is a nonprofit corporation, providing nonmedical, home palliative services on a 7-day-per-week, 24-hour basis and bereavement follow-up, teaching, social, homemaker, spiritual, and public education services. The program began in September 1976. The unit of care is the patient and family. The population served exceeds 1 million, and all patients are within a 30-mile radius. They currently serve three patients and planned to expand to 15 during 1978. They have 15 volunteers who each undergo a 15-hour training program. Thus far, all patients are admitted as cancer patients, but admission is not restricted to cancer patients. Eighty percent of the patients are between 18 and 64 years, and 20 percent are 65 years or older. The funding consists of private contributions and memorials; they anticipate that they soon will have church and foundation grants.

Hospice Buffalo, Inc., Buffalo, New York. A nonprofit corporation program begun in 1975, it is composed entirely of lay volunteers who provide teaching and instruction through a public awareness campaign. They provide speakers to organizations and public gatherings, espousing the philosophy of hospice. They have 220 volunteers in the program, 20 of whom are active. Each of the actives provide 5 hours' service per week after undergoing a ten-week, 2½-hour-per-week training session. Thus, there are 2.5 full-time equivalent volunteers in the program. They planned to provide home care within Erie County by the fall of 1978. Inpatient care is pending New York State licensure and site availability.

Hospice Care of Mid-America, Kansas City, Missouri. This is a nonprofit group that presently sees patients through an outpatient clinic. They have tendered an offer to buy an extended-care facility, and they plan to use 20 currently empty beds for hospice care. Thus, they will provide inpatient and outpatient palliative care as well as consulting and referral, bereavement follow-up, teaching, counseling, spiritual, and social services. Their program began in September 1977. The normal visiting times will be six days per week, 24 hours per day, with no age restrictions. The unit of care is the patient and family. They serve a population of greater than 1 million, and all the patients come from within a ten-mile radius. They serve four home care patients through telephone contact and hospital emergency room back-up. They have 25 volunteers who each provide two hours' service per week after three three-hour training sessions, including a home visit. Full-time equivalent personnel: RN, 0.20; social worker, 0.20; physician, 0.25; clergy, 0.50; administrative, 0.20. All the patients are cancer patients, 75 percent between the ages of 18 and 64, and 25 percent aged 65 and over. They have no funding at present, and they do not charge patients.

Hospice of Marin, Kentfield, California. A nonprofit corporation providing home care and consulting and referral, bereavement follow-up, teaching, counseling, homemaker, spiritual, art therapy, and social services, their program began in February 1976. The unit of care is the patient and the family. They serve a population base of up to 500,000, with all the patients residing within 30 miles of the office. They provide home care services seven days per week, 24 hours per day, and they can serve between 25 and 30 patients. They have 30 professional volunteers providing patient care plus 40 members of an auxiliary called "Friends of Hospice." Each volunteer provides eight hours' service per week. All volunteers attend an information meeting; the professionals also attend a weekly patient care conference. No lay volunteers are used in patient care. All the patients are cancer patients. The revenue is totally philanthropic: foundations, 52 percent; organizations, 7 percent; memorial donations, 27 percent; individual donations, 10 percent; interest and miscellaneous, 4 percent.

Hospice of the Monterey Peninsula, Carmel, California. A program that began in April 1976, it provides home palliative, consulting and referral, bereavement follow-up, teaching, counseling, spiritual, and social services. They were scheduled to have opened a six-bed, inpatient palliative care unit in the Spring of 1978. Visiting is allowed seven days per week and 24 hours per day, with no age restrictions. The unit of care is the patient and the family. The population served is up to 500,000, with all patients coming from within a 30-mile radius. Home care is provided seven days per week, 24 hours per day. There are 40 volunteers who each provide about 18 hours' service per month and receive 25 hours of class instruction and subsequently 10 hours of inservice training. Full-time equivalent personnel: RN, 3; LVN, 4; social worker, 1; physician, 0.5;

administrative, 2; housekeeping, 1; program coordinator, 2. Ninety-eight percent of the patients are cancer patients and 2 percent are heart patients; 2 percent are under 18, 80 percent are between 18 and 64, and 18 percent are 65 and over. They are negotiating with the State Department of Health to be classified as an intermediate nursing facility. Funding comes from foundation, county, memorial, and general donations, from the American Cancer Society, and from self-paying patients. They plan to allow patients' families to stay at their inpatient facility.

Hospice Orange County, Inc., Laguna Hills, California. A nonprofit corporation whose program began in August 1977, it offers inpatient palliative care (through a local hospital and a convalescent facility), home palliative care, and consulting and referral, bereavement follow-up, counseling, homemaker, spiritual, teaching, and social services. There are no visitor age restrictions, and visiting is allowed seven days per week, 24 hours per day. The unit of care is the patient and family. The population served is up to 500,000, with all patients coming from within a 30-mile radius. Home care is provided seven days per week, 24 hours per day. They serve 20 patients, and the average length of stay is ten days. There are 50 volunteers in the program, with professionals providing six hours' service per week and lay volunteers providing 3 hours' service per week. All personnel are volunteer except the coordinator, who is salaried at 24 hours per week. All patients are cancer patients; 90 percent are between the ages of 18 and 64, and 10 percent are 65 or over. Except for physician home visits, the hospice operates entirely through volunteer services. Inpatient beds (by arrangement) are provided only when it becomes impossible to care for the patient at home. For overnight stays, the hospital supplies a rollaway bed in the patient's room and, when space is available, a private room for other family members or friends.

Hospice Orlando, Inc., Orlando, Florida. This is a nonprofit corporation whose program began in October 1976. They currently provide home care and consulting and referral, bereavement follow-up, counseling, teaching, homemaker, spiritual, and social services. They are expecting to provide an inpatient facility in the future. The population served is between 500,000 and 1 million, and all of the patients are within a 30-mile radius of the office. Home care services are provided seven days per week, 24 hours per day for between 25 and 30 patients. There are 25 volunteers who each provide ten hours' service per week after undergoing training consisting of a one-day seminar and several visits with an experienced volunteer; ongoing training is also provided. There is one part-time (16 hours per week) paid nurse. All others are volunteers. All patients are cancer patients; 52 percent are between 18 and 64, and 48 percent are aged 65 and over. Funding is from church donations, the American Cancer

Society, private donations, and memorials. Patients are not charged, except for the services of the medical director, who sees patients on a consulting basis and bills as a private physician.

Hospice of Salt Lake, Inc., Salt Lake City, Utah. A nonprofit corporation, it provides home care, inpatient palliative care, and consulting and referral, bereavement follow-up, teaching, counseling, spiritual, and social services. The program began in December 1977. The patient and family are the unit of care. The population served is between 500,000 and 1 million, and all patients come from within a 30-mile radius of the office. They provide home care services seven days per week, 24 hours per day. Seven home care patients are served by 40 professional volunteers and 7 lay volunteers, who provide three hours' service per day. Volunteers undergo the following training: selection, cardiopulmonary resuscitation, psychology, and body mechanics. All the staff are volunteers. All patients are cancer patients, 50 percent between 18 and 64, and 50 percent aged 65 and over. Funding comes from foundations and private donations. No overnight accommodations are provided for patients' families.

Hospice of Santa Barbara, Inc., Santa Barbara, California. This nonprofit corporation provides inpatient palliative care (through Pinecrest Hospital), home care, and consulting and referral, bereavement follow-up, teaching, youth group, counseling, homemaker, spiritual, and social services. The program began in December 1974. The unit of care is the patient and family. The population served is approximately 225,000; 50 patients are served. Three chapters are located in the county under one administrative head. Services are provided to anyone regardless of age or financial status; no fee is charged. Care is coordinated with other community service programs, including Visiting Nurses, County Social Service, the County Medical Society, and pharmacological organizations. Approximately 65 volunteers donate about ten hours' service per week after attending mandatory eight-week classes plus ongoing monthly training classes. Full-time equivalent personnel: social worker, 1, physician, 0.50; administrative, 2; secretarial, 1. The patients are admitted to the program with diagnoses of cancer (70 percent), heart disease (10 percent), and arteriosclerosis (20 percent); 35 percent are between 18 and 64, and 65 percent are 65 and over. Funding sources include a Presbyterian Church grant, a grant from the Area Agency on Aging, the American Cancer Society, city and county revenue sharing, and one CETA position.

Hospice of Solano, Vallejo, California. A nonprofit organization whose incorporation is pending, it provides home care, consulting and referral, bereavement follow-up, teaching, counseling, homemaker, spiritual, and social services. Their program began in June 1977, and they do not anticipate planning for a hospice facility. The patient and the family are the unit of care. The population base served is between 100,000 and 500,000. The home care services are provided through public and private agencies for a maximum of five days per week. The organization is almost totally volunteer, with professional volunteers providing five hours' service per week each, and nonprofessionals providing 15. All volunteers receive continuing training. Patients are admitted to the program with the following diagnoses: cancer (75 percent), kidney disease (10 percent), heart disease (10 percent), and old age (5 percent); 75 percent of the patients are between 18 and 64, and 25 percent are 65 and over. Funding is provided 50 percent through memberships, memorials, and donations, and 50 percent through a grant from the North Bay Senior Planning Council, Area V.

Lutheran Medical Center, Continuing Care Unit, Saint Louis, Missouri. A nonprofit corporation that began its program on January 9, 1978, it has a 12-bed, inpatient palliative care unit, and provides home palliative care, consulting and referral, counseling, spiritual, teaching, and social services as well as music therapy and physical therapy. There are no age restrictions for visitors and visiting is allowed seven days per week, 24 hours per day. The unit of care is the patient and family. The population served is greater than 1 million, with patients coming from the following estimated distances: less than 10 miles (50 percent), 10 to 30 miles (25 percent), 30 to 49 miles (25 percent). Home care services are provided five days per week, 8:00 A.M. to 4:30 P.M., with emergency on-call. The average length of stay for inpatients is 8.5 days; the average daily patient census is six. Fifteen volunteers each provide three hours' service per week, after a three-session orientation plus ongoing inservice. Full-time equivalent personnel: RN, 8; LPN, 5; social worker, 1.5; physician, 1; clergy, 1; administrative, 2; housekeeping, 1. About 90 percent of the patients are admitted with cancer diagnoses, and 10 percent with kidney disorders; 45 percent are between 18 and 64, and 55 percent are 65 and over. Funding comes primarily from foundations, church support, and the Lutheran Charities Association. Patients' families are accommodated in three rooms furnished with living room furniture, day beds, and/or hide-a-beds.

Methodist Hospital, Hospice Unit, Indianapolis, Indiana. This nonprofit hospital has an 11-bed inpatient unit that provides home care, bereavement follow-up, teaching, counseling, spiritual, and social services. The program began in July 1977. There are no age restrictions for visitors, who may visit seven days per week, 24 hours per day. The patient and family plus "significant others" are the unit of care. The population served is between 500,000 and 1 million, with patients coming from the following distances: less than 10 miles (79 percent), 10 to 29 miles (7 percent), 30 to 49 miles (2 percent), and 50 to 100 miles (12 percent). Home care is provided only via telephone from unit personnel and visits by commercial agencies. They are not planning to provide any further home care services. The average daily inpatient census is nine; the average length of stay is 11.9 days. There are 21 volunteers in the program who each provide three hours of service per week. Each volunteer gets 10 to 12 hours' training, with follow-up, on-the-unit training on the buddy system. Full-time equivalent personnel: RN, 9; LPN, 3; community health liaison nurse, 1; nursing assistants, 3. Admitting diagnoses of patients are cancer (98 percent) and amyotrophic lateral sclerosis (2 percent). Seventy percent of the patients are between 18 and 64, and 30 percent are 65 and over. For third-party reimbursement, the 11 beds are classified as acute hospital beds. All revenue comes from a combination of Medicare, Medicaid, commercial insurance, and self-pay. There are no special overnight accommodations for patients' families.

Midpeninsula Health Service, Inc., Home Care Department, Palo Alto, California. This nonprofit corporation began its program in February 1977. It provides home palliative care, consulting and referral, bereavement follow-up, teaching, nursing, counseling, homemaker, lay volunteer, and social services. Caregivers normally visit the home five days (40 hours) per week and are on call 24 hours per day, 7 days per week. The unit of care is the patient and the family. The population served is less than 100,000. They serve 10 to 20 patients simultaneously. Ten lay volunteers are involved in the program. Each of the volunteers participates in a complete workshop that includes communication and "many aspects of health care." Full-time equivalent personnel: RN, 2; social worker, 1; physician, 1; administrative, 1; housekeeping, 0.5; home health aide, 0.5. Patients are admitted to program with diagnoses of cancer (40 percent), kidney disease (2 percent), heart disease (32 percent), and "various diseases" (2 percent). Two percent of the patients are under 18 years of age, 22 percent are between 18 and 64, and 76 percent are 65 and over. Revenue comes from Medicare (84 percent), commercial insurance (10 percent), and self-pay (6 percent). Funding is primarily from private foundations and member dues.

National In-Home Health Services, Van Nuys, California. This investor-owned corporation's program began informally in November 1976 and was formalized in September 1977. It provides home palliative care, consulting and referral, counseling, nursing, lay volunteer, teaching, social, and nutritional and pharmaceutical consultation services; it also "informally" provides bereavement follow-up services. The patients served are from a population base of greater than 1,000,000. Patients come from the following distances: less than 10 miles (35 percent), 10 to 30 miles (55 percent), and 30 to 50 miles (10 percent). The home care services are provided during days seven days per week, with phone service for nights. The patient load is unlimited. Full-time equivalent personnel: RN, 13.5; LPN, 1; social worker, 1.5; administrative, 4; home health aides, 7; physical therapist, 3; occupational therapist, 1. Patients are admitted to the program with following diagnoses: cancer (75 percent), heart disease (20 percent), and respiratory disease (5 percent). One percent of the patients are under 18 years of age, 24 percent are between 18 and 64, and 75 percent are 65 and older. Revenue sources are Medicare (95 percent), Medicaid (2 percent), and commercial insurance (3 percent). These are the only sources of funding.

Overlook Hospital, Summit, New Jersey. This 551-bed, nonprofit corporation community and teaching hospital provides no inpatient hospice services. It does provide home palliative care, consulting and referral, bereavement follow-up, teaching, counseling, homemaker, social, nutritional counseling, occupational, physical therapy, and spiritual and emotional group services. The program began in January 1977. The patient and family are the unit of care. All patients are from within a 30-mile area consisting of the 11 municipalities comprising the hospital's service area, and the population served is between 100,000 and 500,000. Home care services are provided 24 hours per day, seven days per week. The maximum daily number of home care patients who can be accommodated is 40. There are currently nine trained volunteers who each provide 1½ hours service daily, and whose training consists of six intensive training sessions. Full-time equivalent personnel: RN, 7; LPN, 1; social worker, 0.3; physician, 0.1; clergy, 0.1; administrative, 0.2. All patients are admitted with a cancer diagnosis. Forty-nine percent are between 18 and 64, and 51 percent are 65 and over. Revenue comes from Medicare (51 percent), commercial insurance (40 percent), self-pay (1 percent), and Blue Cross (8 percent); additional funding is provided by foundations and personal contributions. No overnight accommodations are provided for patients' families.

Parkwood Community Hospital, Hospice Unit, Canoga Park, California. This investor-owned corporation hospice began in October 1976. It consists of a 14-bed inpatient palliative care program offering consulting and referral, bereavement follow-up, teaching, counseling, spiritual, and social services. Visiting is permitted 24 hours per day, seven days per week, with no age restrictions. The unit of care is the patient and family, and sometimes a nonfamily "important person" may be added. The population base served is greater than 1 million. Home care services are provided only through existing community nursing and social agencies. They are planning to coordinate these agencies better to provide outpatient hospice-level care. The average length of inpatient stay is about 12 to 14 days, with an average daily census of five to seven. About 12 volunteers are involved, rendering an average of 6 hours' service per week after preservice orientation. Full-time equivalent personnel: RN, 4.8; LVN, 1.6; social worker, 1.0; administrative, 1.0; housekeeping, 0.5; others, 3.0; physician services provided by private practitioners. Patients are admitted with diagnoses of cancer (99 percent) and amyotrophic lateral sclerosis (1 percent). The inpatient beds are classified as acute hospital beds for third-party reimbursement purposes. Revenue comes from Medicare (31.5 percent), Medicaid (9.9 percent), commercial insurance (48.8 percent), and other (9.8 percent). Special overnight accommodations for patients' families can occasionally be provided in the family room or in patients' rooms.

Pinecrest Hospital, Santa Barbara, California. This program provides inpatient palliative care through its 24-bed unit and through consulting and referral, bereavement and follow-up, counseling, spiritual, and social services. They work closely with Hospice of Santa Barbara, Inc., getting inpatient referrals from that organization. The program began in January 1975. There are no visitor age restrictions, and visiting is permitted seven days per week, 24 hours per day. The unit of care is the patient, family, and friends. The population served is about 225,000. Patients coming from less than 10 miles represent 30 percent of all patients, those from 10 to 30 miles represent 60 percent, those from 30 to 50 miles represent 8 percent, and those from 50 to 100 miles represent 2 percent. The average daily inpatient census is 20; the average length of stay is 18 days. Between 10 and 12 volunteers are in the program, and each provides two hours' service weekly. The admitting diagnoses of patients are cancer (90 percent), kidney disease (2 percent), heart disease (6 percent), and neurological diseases (2 percent). Twenty percent of the patients are between 18 and 64, and 80 percent are 65 and over. Revenue comes from Medicare (80 percent), commercial insurance (19 percent), and self-pay (1 percent). Special overnight accommodations of patients' families consists of two lounge chairs, one couch, and, if available, a hospital bed. The patient beds are classified both as acute hospital beds and, in an adjacent unit, as skilled nursing facility beds.

Riverside Hospice, Boonton, New Jersey. This nonprofit division of Riverside Hospital was begun in January 1977. It offers home palliative care, consulting and referral, bereavement follow-up, teaching, counseling, spiritual, and social services. In April 1978, a 16-bed unit for inpatient palliative care was scheduled to have been added. The patient and family are the unit of care. The patients from 30 miles' distance represent 80 percent of all patients, the remaining 20 percent coming from as far away as 50 miles. They provide home care services 24 hours a day, seven days per week, and they can serve up to 50 patients. Ninety volunteers are involved in the program. Each receives a ten-week, 20-hour course and a minimum additional six-hour practicum. Full-time equivalent personnel: RN and LPN, "changing"; social worker, 0.5; physician, 1.0; clergy, 0.25; administrative, 2.0; housekeeping, 1.5; educator, 1.0; psychologist, 0.25. All patients have an admitting diagnosis of cancer; half are between the ages of 18 and 64, and half are 65 and over. Funding comes from foundations, federal grants, and the state government. The hospice is supported by the National Cancer Institute (NCI) Contract No. 1 CN-75391, except for the educator, whose cost is supported by a grant from the New Jersey Department of Health.

Rogers Memorial Hospital, Oconomowoc, Wisconsin. This hospice unit of ten beds began operations on January 15, 1978. It is a nonprofit, nonstock corporation providing inpatient palliative care, home palliative care, consulting and referral, bereavement follow-up, teaching, counseling, spiritual, and social services. Visiting is permitted 24 hours per day, seven days per week, with no age restrictions. The patient and family are the unit of care. The unit serves a populaticn of over 1 million. Home care services for 35 patients are provided on a 24-hour, seven-day basis. Inpatient average length of stay is expected to be about 14 days. Approximately 50 volunteers are involved, each giving three hours' service per week. After initial screening, each volunteer receives ten hours of orientation. Full-time equivalent personnel: RN, 4.2; LPN, 4.2; social worker, 1.0; physician, 4.0; clergy, 0.75; administrative, 1.5, housekeeping, 2.0; home care coordinator, 1.0; head nurse, 1.0. The unit is classified as psychiatric for third-party reimbursement purposes. The revenue breakdown is Medicare/Medicaid, 21 percent; commercial insurance, 51 percent; and self-pay, 28 percent. Some foundation funding is available. Overnight accommodations for patients' families is provided by means of three private rooms with half-baths across from patient rooms. The facility is located on 76 wooded acres with two lakes and with trails for hiking.

St. John's Hospital (Mercy Hospice), Oxnard, California. This nonprofit organization began its clinical operations in July 1976. It provides home palliative care, consulting and referral, bereavement follow-up, teaching, counseling, partial homemaker, spiritual, and social services. It is a field placement facility for seminary students. The hospice has worked with all hospital oncology cases, the average daily census of which is 15. A two-bed hospice inpatient unit was expected to have been operational by May 1978. There are no age restrictions for visitors, who are welcome 24 hours per day, seven days per week. The unit of care is the patient and family. The population served is less than 100,000, with all patients coming from within a 20-mile radius. About 20 to 30 home care patients are served 24 hours per day, seven days per week. The oncology inpatients average a 14-day length of stay. Currently, there are six trained volunteers, with an additional 20 in training. Each volunteer provides a minimum of six hours' service per week after a concentrated training program is completed. Full-time equivalent personnel: RN, 1.5; social worker, 0.5; clergy, 0.25; administrative, 0.5; secretary, 0.5. Admitting diagnoses of patients are cancer (95 percent) and pulmonary diseases (5 percent). Ten percent of the patients are under 18 years of age, 70 percent are between 18 and 64 years, and 20 percent are 65 and older. The beds are classified as both acute hospital and skilled nursing beds. Revenue comes from Medicare (85 percent), Medicaid (10 percent), and commercial insurance (5 percent). There are limited overnight accommodations for patients' families; about one person per patient can be accommodated.

St. Michael's Hospital Palliative Care Programme, Toronto, Ontario, Canada. This program is hospitalwide, including all 750 of the hospital's active acute treatment beds. The hospital is owned and administered by the religious community. The program has provided inpatient palliative care, consulting and referral, teaching, spiritual, and social services since May 1977. There are no age restrictions for visitors. The unit of care is the patient and family. The hospital does not provide home care services but uses community resources, up to eight hours per day, five days per week. A small group of six to eight volunteers is being trained to be involved in patient and family care. Full-time equivalent personnel: RN, 1.0; physician, 0.4. Additionally, specially trained multidisciplinary teams function on each nursing unit. The patients' admitting diagnoses are cancer (96 percent), and heart disease (4 percent). Eighty percent are between 18 and 64, and 20 percent are 65 and over. Funding is provided by the Ontario provincial government. No overnight accommodations are provided for patients' families.

San Diego County Hospice Corporation, San Diego, California. This nonprofit corporation's program began in October 1977 and provides home palliative care, consulting and referral, bereavement follow-up, teaching, counseling, homemaker, and spiritual services. Home care services are provided 24 hours per day, seven days per week for about 30 patients per year. The service population is greater than 1 million, and all patients come from within a 10-mile radius. Twenty volunteers each provide about two hours' service per week; they receive eight two-hour training sessions followed by bimonthly inservice training. All patients are cancer patients, and their ages are evenly divided between the 18-to-64 age group and the 65-and-over group. All revenue is derived from foundation philanthropy. No overnight accommodations are provided for patients' families.

West Hills Hospital, Canoga Park, California. This program is a 32-bed oncology unit of an investor-owned corporation acute hospital. It provides inpatient palliative care, consulting and referral, bereavement follow-up, teaching, counseling, homemaker (via agencies), spiritual, and social services. The program has been in operation since March 1977. There are no age restrictions for visitors, and visiting is permitted 24 hours per day, seven days per week. The unit of care is the patient and family. The population base served is 500,000 to 1 million, and all patients come from up to 30 miles' distance. No home care is provided except for telephone consultation and outside agency services. Home care services are planned for the future. The average daily inpatient census is ten. The average length of stay is 14 to 21 days. There are four volunteers, who each provide four to five hours' service per day. Full-time equivalent personnel: RN, 5; LVN, 1; social worker, 1; physician, 3; administrative, 1; housekeeping, 2; nurses' assistant, 3. All patients are admitted with cancer diagnoses; 40 percent are between 18 and 64, and 60 percent are 65 and over. Revenue comes from Medicare (60 percent), Medicaid (20 percent), and commercial insurance (20 percent). Special overnight accommodations for families of patients are provided. Additionally, a special family room is available in which the patient may entertain.

Hospices in Planning Stages

A total of 23 hospices were identified as being in various stages of planning. Some respondents replied with short letters indicating that since they were only in the preliminary planning stages, they could offer no responses to the questionnaire. Others attempted to complete the questionnaire as best they could, guessing at many questions or omitting answers entirely. Following is an alphabetical listing of each respondent who gave permission to use the information, with a summary of pertinent information.

Ad Hoc Hospice Committee, Claremont, California. The Pilgrim Place Medical Center (McCabe Rest Home) provides hospice-type care in certain situations. They have an architect working on drawings for a new health center that will house a hospice program. Currently, they are only a committee meeting on an ad hoc basis.

The Burke Rehabilitation Center, White Plains, New York. The master plan for the hospice includes a new day hospital, apartments for physically handicapped and mentally alert adults, and a skilled nursing and health-related facility.

The Elisabeth Kubler-Ross Hospice, Inc., Clearwater, Florida. This program was expected to have begun in April 1978. It ultimately will involve five facilities, each with about 15 beds. In addition to the customary hospice-type services, they will offer legal and financial consulting. They expect that 99 percent of all patients will be admitted with cancer diagnoses. About 90 percent of the patients are expected to be 65 or over. They expect the facilities to be classified as "special hospital" facilities for third-party reimbursement purposes. They expect that 50 percent of revenues will come from Medicare, 5 percent from self-pay, and 45 percent from philanthropy. They expect to provide overnight family accommodations in the patients' rooms.

El Cajon Valley Hospital, El Cajon, California. This program was expected to have started in late February 1978. It will provide a four-bed inpatient unit but no home care services. They plan to have day beds or sleeper sofas for overnight family accommodations.

Fairview Community Hospitals, Minneapolis, Minnesota. They planned to have opened their program by around May 1978. Three hospitals owned corporately will have 30 acute inpatient beds and will offer home care 24 hours per day, seven days per week. They expect to have 40 volunteers, each providing two hours' service per week. They expect all patients will have cancer diagnoses. They anticipate that revenues will come 50 percent from Medicare, 20 percent from Medicaid, and 30 percent from commercial insurance. No overnight patient accommodations will be provided.

Hospice of Humboldt, Arcata, California. In the process of formation as a nonprofit corporation, they are undecided whether they will provide hospice services strictly on a home care basis or whether an existing, long-term care facility will be used. They indicated that they would not be ready to deliver services before late 1978.

Hospice of North Carolina, Inc., Winston-Salem, North Carolina. This program was expected to have begun around November or December 1978. They expect to provide both inpatient and home care palliative service plus all the usual hospice services. This organization is unique in that it is a statewide organization; they expect to develop local hospice "chapters," to be supported and encouraged by the corporate offices. The chapters will be the actual providers of hospice inpatient and home care.

Hospice of North Texas, Incorporated, Dallas, Texas. Expected to have been operational by July 1978. They expect to have a 50-bed inpatient unit and 24-hour-per-day, seven-day-per-week home care services. In addition to the usual hospice services, they expect to offer a day-care center and funeral and estate planning. There will be unlimited visiting, including pets. Patients will come from a radius of up to 100 miles, with 80 percent coming from between 30 and 50 miles. Patient family accommodations will be provided at on-site units or through arrangements worked out with local motels.

Hospice of San Francisco, San Francisco, California. Their six-month planning period was funded by the San Francisco Foundation and the planning firm, Gerontological Planning Associates. A report and recommendations were expected around May 1978.

Hospice of San Luis Obispo County, Avila Beach, California. Home care services, but not inpatient palliative care, will be provided with the usual hospice services. Additionally, children's services will be offered. The program was expected to have begun July or August 1978.

Hospice of Tulare County, Tulare, California. They plan to provide all usual hospice services, including inpatient and home care palliative services. They are still a study group offering community education but are expanding into a larger interdisciplinary committee to develop a permanent organization.

Kaiser-Permanente Medical Care Program, Los Angeles, California. The program was expected to have begun by the middle of 1978, offering inpatient and home care palliative services in addition to the usual hospice services. They will have a 15-bed unit and will be able to serve about 35 home care patients. They are planning to provide overnight family accommodations.

Long Beach Community Hospital, Long Beach, California. The program was expected to have begun in the fall of 1978. They will provide a 16-bed inpatient unit and expect to provide home care services 24 hours per day, seven days per week. Patients are expected to come from within 30 miles, with 95 percent coming from within less than 10 miles. Cancer patients will make up 98 percent of the admissions, and beds will be provided by the hospital for families.

Our Lady of Lourdes Memorial Hospital, Binghamton, New York. The hospice is not yet operational, but consultation services are provided to dying patients and their families.

St. Agnes Hospice (St. Agnes Medical Center), Fresno, California. The program was to have begun sometime during 1978. All the customary hospice services, including inpatient and home palliative care, will be provided, the latter on a 24-hour-per-day, seven-day-per-week basis. There will be no visiting restrictions. To implement the program, existing personnel, who also have other hospital duties, will be utilized in the hospice unit.

St. Clare's Mercy Hospital, St. John's, Newfoundland, Canada. They are in the early stages of planning a small, 12-bed unit for palliative care, as a special-care unit of the 340-bed general hospital.

St. Mary's Hospital, Richmond, Virginia. They are in the very early phase of planning.

San Francisco Regional Cancer Foundation, San Francisco, California. See Hospice San Francisco.

The Southeast Texas Hospice, Orange, Texas. The program was expected to have been operational by April or May 1978. They expect to provide a 24-bed inpatient unit, home care services on a 24-hour-per-day, seven-day-per-week basis, and all the customary hospice services. Additionally, the hospice will be a state demonstration center for research on pain. They have applied to the Texas Health Facilities Commission for a certificate of need for the home care program as a home health agency. They claim to be the first hospice in Texas.

Visiting Nurse Association, Inc. Serving Alameda County, Oakland, California. They don't profess to be a hospice but are a licensed home health agency. They could assume the home care aspects and are planning to develop a preplanned, 24-hour call service for patients requiring nursing services at home at other than the regularly scheduled hours. They are developing special cancer care teams made up of multidisciplinary team members. Partial funding for this project was provided by the American Cancer Society.

Washington Hospice Society, Inc., Washington, D.C. They are planning to provide all hospice services, including a 40-bed, free-standing facility, if possible. This program is just in the preliminary planning stages, but 350 volunteers are potentially available.

Anonymous Program, Illinois. This program should have been operational in May 1978. It will provide customary hospice services, including an inpatient unit of possibly six beds. The unit of care will be the patient, family, and extended family. Ninety percent of all patients are expected to come from within a radius of 10 to 30 miles and from a population base of less than 100,000. Admitting diagnoses are expected to be cancer (80 percent), kidney disease (5 percent), and heart disease (15 percent).

Anonymous Program, California. At present, this is strictly a volunteer program, currently labeled "Patient Support Program." Planning has three phases: 1) pilot project giving service to a small number of patients (task-oriented services are grocery shopping, sitting with patient, chauffeuring, food preparation, etc.); 2) more involvement with patients and families, including more direct emotional support and counseling; 3) final, hospital-based hospice, incorporating the experiences of phases 1 and 2 and the hospital's oncology department and home care service.

Community Support Group-Hospice Concept

This organization in Menlo Park, California is a loosely affiliated group of professionals and volunteers who meet monthly for continuing education, communication, and moral support. They are interested in the creation of hospice-type services within the existing health care system. They have no plans for this group to be anything more than a forum.

SUMMARY AND CONCLUSIONS

The respondents to the questionnaire included representatives of each of the following hospice models: the freestanding unit, hospital hospice unit, the hospital-wide hospice with a moving multidisciplinary team serving hospice patients anywhere in the hospital, the hospital oncology unit, the home care program, the day care program, the community support group, the all-volunteer group (both professionals and lay volunteers), those organizations that charged patients, and those that levied no charges to patients.

The "typical" hospice model represented by the survey is a nonprofit corporation offering home palliative care, inpatient palliative care (either through their own facility's beds or through an arrangement with a local hospital or convalescent home), consulting and referral, bereavement follow-up, medical and nursing, counseling, spiritual, teaching, and social services. Visiting hours and days are unlimited, with no age restrictions for visitors. The patient and family are the unit of care. The great bulk of the patients come from within a 30-mile radius, and the population base served is about 500,000. Home care services are provided seven days per week, 24 hours per day for about 35 patients. The average length of stay for inpatients is about 14 days. There are about 30 volunteers in the program, who each contribute about four hours' service per week after about 20 hours of orientation and inservice training. The numbers of personnel are extremely varied, and no generalizations can be made; however, usually a team is used consisting of the following disciplines: registered nurse, licensed vocational/practical nurse, social worker, physician, clergy, administrative personnel, and nursing assistants. The overwhelming number of patients are admitted with cancer diagnoses. More than half the patients are 65 years or older; only about 5 percent are under 18 years of age. Most of the inpatient beds are classified as acute hospital beds. Funding and revenues come from foundations, federal grants, state government, philanthropy, commercial insurance, Medicare, and Medicaid. Some accommodations are provided for overnight stay of patients' families.

In Appendix A will be found a listing, compiled after the hospice survey, of more than 250 hospices in the British Isles, Canada, and the United States. This listing by no means should be considered complete, since new groups are continually forming and at the present time there is no central reporting or licensing agency for hospices.

Chapter 12

Roadblocks to the Hospice Movement

Many things difficult to design prove easy to performance.
Samuel Johnson, *Rasselas*

At present, there are several roadblocks to hospice development, and once the design is completed (or, in our case, more aptly, once the roadblocks are removed), the performance will become easy. Most of these roadblocks, or obstacles, stem from attitudes—attitudes of legislators, bureaucrats, health professionals, fiscal intermediaries and health insurance policy makers, and society at large.

In May 1977, the Third National Hospice Symposium was presented at the Dominican College Campus in San Rafael, California. The listing of nine major obstacles to hospice development that was presented at this symposium is included here as a frame of reference.

1. *The hospice idea.* Problems are created by the fact that death and dying is a taboo subject that arouses many personal and cultural fears.
2. *Ignorance of the hospice care process.* Education is needed.
   - General public—frequent community presentations
   - Physicians—education and persuasion rather than criticism; accent on symptom control, team approach, and consultation rather than takeover of patients
   - Other health care professionals (nurses, psychologists, physical therapists, dieticians, etc.)—accent on the special needs of the terminally ill
   - Other health organizations—determination of who does what; avoidance of duplication of services; maintenance of hospice organizations' autonomy
   - The media—education to combat their cynicism, biases, and tendency toward sensationalism
3. *The need for money.* Too little money can threaten hospice's existence; improperly used money can destroy its integrity.

4. *Regulatory agencies*. We must educate agencies and be prepared for frequent presentations/public hearings. They may grant assistance to a new "hospice" category in some states.
5. *Statutes and regulations*. As the hospice movement develops, licensure and third-party payment questions arise.
6. *The euthanasia issue*. We must distinguish hospice from euthanasia. There is real danger of equating the two.
7. *The internal environment*. Our own hangups and procrastinations can cause us trouble. A can-do attitude is necessary.
8. *Organizational structure*. We need the ability to change as the need changes. There are many volunteer aspects to this type of care.
9. *The team need*. The recruitment, selection, training, and integration of a team are all very necessary. It must work effectively together for the patient and family.[1]

THE HOSPICE IDEA

Death evokes many fears; consequently, many refuse to acknowledge death, particularly their own deaths. Their attitude seems to be, "If I ignore it, maybe it will disappear. It's too bad about John dying last week, but it can't happen to me (or it will happen so far in the future, why should I be concerned now). I am immortal. I feel healthy. If I put the idea of death out of mind, maybe I won't ever have to experience it."

Yet, though death has been a taboo topic for many years, people are now being exposed more and more to discussions on death and dying. Self-help groups for cancer patients and the bereaved, community discussion groups, workshops and seminars have begun to proliferate in recent years. The hospice method of caring for the terminally ill is beginning to catch on, but much work needs to be done in spreading the hospice idea.

The overwhelming majority of people, when faced with the need to care for terminally ill family members look to the acute general hospitals or nursing homes. Although in a great many cases this may be an appropriate approach, in a larger number of cases, it may be less than appropriate.

The hospice idea has been introduced and is beginning to take hold, but as yet it is still a new concept. The next five years are critical. Proper influence of all segments of the public that the hospice industry serves will determine if the hospice idea will spread or if it will die.

IGNORANCE OF THE HOSPICE CARE PROCESS

Generally, the hospice idea is unknown; it is a relatively new concept in the United States. The general public needs to be educated about the hospice care process. This can be accomplished by presentations to the community by hospice practitioners and other interested people, universities, hospice organizations, and others (see Recommendations in Chapter 13).

Many physicians are not aware of the hospice philosophy, and they, too, need to be educated. According to Michael Van Scoy-Mosher, former chairman of the department of oncology at Cedars-Sinai Medical Center, Los Angeles, another problem exists with physicians and the institutionalized hospice patients. He claims it is a matter of geography in that doctors cannot travel long distances to attend to hospice terminal patients in locations remote from the doctors' usual hospital practice.[2] Another possible implicit objection could be that the family physician would "lose" patients and the consequent financial return. Also, Van Scoy-Mosher claims that patients do not wish to change physicians in their last weeks of life. They don't want to be turned over to new physicians, as might be the case in a hospice.[3]

Other health care professionals and paraprofessionals such as nurses, psychologists, physical therapists, pharmacists, dieticians, etc. need to be educated about the special needs of the terminally ill so that their special skills can be most effectively utilized. The training of physicians and these other health care professionals has been deficient in the area of death and dying. However, in recent years thanatological topics have become less taboo than previously, and courses are being introduced in medical schools, nursing schools, and other schools for health professionals, which, in time, will provide better understanding of the death, dying, and hospice concepts.

At present, there is something of an overlap of hospice functions. Many home health agencies provide homemaker and nursing services but may not offer the symptom control and the counseling offered by hospice programs. Many physicians claim that hospice is not new, that hospitals and nursing homes have provided these services all along. Both the physicians who contend this and the institutions that agree with them are correct to a point. However, few of these institutions concentrate on *caring* for terminally ill patients rather than trying to *cure* them.

The hospice organization needs to be autonomous. Separately or conjointly, it can provide home care, a day-care support center, and inpatient beds, all coordinated with existing community resources.

Although the media can be a tremendous educational asset, it has tended toward sensationalism. Because of the lack of knowledge of reporters and editors, stories have been released in newspapers, magazines, and television that all too often reflect the biases and sarcasm of the authors.

THE NEED FOR MONEY

Capital is needed to build hospice organizations. Hospice requires very little technology, and new buildings are not needed. However, funds are needed to attract, train, and pay hospice personnel and to pay for necessary overhead. Many developing hospices, lacking sufficient seed money, will organize volunteers, both professional and lay, who provide their services at no cost for a period of months. Gradually, money will trickle in in the form of memorials to deceased patients from members of their families. Soon, many hospices find that they are eligible for small grants from communities, private foundations, church groups, etc. As their treasuries grow, some of the key personnel are paid on a limited basis.

As their organizational expertise expands with their experience in caring for the dying and their families, the fledgling hospice organization may find that it can negotiate individually with private insurance carriers, Medicare and Medicaid fiscal intermediaries, and other third-party payers for at least partial reimbursement of hospice expenses.

Yes, money is needed. Too little will threaten the existence of hospices; and money improperly used will threaten the credibility of hospices as providers of necessary health care, leading ultimately to their demise. The capital funds for hospice development are in short supply. The concept is still relatively new, and investors can find suitable investment vehicles with considerably less risk attached that practically assure a positive return on investments. No such assurance exists today for hospice investment. As one study found, "establishment of a hospice would be a relatively high risk venture at this time."[4]

REGULATORY AGENCIES

At this writing, no states have regulations covering hospice care. Hospices, therefore, are hybrids. They are neither hospitals nor nursing homes, and many are not home health agencies. Yet they may be functioning as parts of all three types of organizations. Until the question of licensure categories is determined by individual states, regulatory agencies will have very little to regulate. Statutes must first be enacted by the states to provide legal backgrounds and frames of reference from which the regulatory bodies *then* can prepare regulations and licensing codes with which hospices can be held accountable.

At present, we have almost a free-for-all hospice development and existence. This free enterprise approach may not be bad, however. Experience has shown that when government interferes with private enterprise, costs escalate, delays hinder development, and the public suffers.

The creation of additional levels of bureaucracy would have the inevitable effect of hindering hospice development.

Do hospices need to be licensed? What advantages can be gained that are not now available under our present free enterprise system? Probably the most important answer to that question relates to reimbursement. Many third-party payers reimburse based on the definition of the health provider as set out in the various state health and welfare codes. No definition, no (or little) reimbursement. Hence, licensing is essential. William Lamers advocates a licensing category called "hospice care," which he feels would open the way for reimbursement of psychological, spiritual, and emotional support.[5]

Although the National Cancer Institute has circulated requests for proposals (RFPs) for free-standing hospices[6] and three awards have been made,[7] it appears unlikely that free-standing hospices will become the mode of development. The future of hospices in this country could become linked to the number of unused acute-care beds.[8] With occupancy rates of acute-care beds declining in recent years, these beds might be considered "excess" for acute care, but not for hospice care. Caution must be exerted to prevent conversion of these beds to hospice use as an attempt to disguise inappropriate maintenance of excess acute-care beds.[9]

Hospice needs to be considered in current health care planning. The health systems agencies under the aegis of the National Health Planning and Resources Development Act of 1974 (PL 93-641) must take into consideration the special needs of the terminally ill and their families. At the moment, planning for hospices is almost nonexistent. This is so, again, primarily because of the lack of hospice knowledge among the general public and health systems agency members.

When the public becomes aware of hospice, then the legislators will react. A public groundswell in favor of hospice can have a decided effect on legislators; positive public sentiment will accelerate legislation, licensing, and consequent reimbursement policies.

THE EUTHANASIA ISSUE

Hospice is not euthanasia. Hospice is a caring community of care givers, dedicated to providing comfort and loving care to terminally ill people and their families. Their aim is to ease the final weeks, days, and hours of a person's life—to cushion that journey toward the final rest.

On the other hand, euthanasia means "an easy death"—action (or inaction) that most probably will result in the patient's death. Giving drugs to hasten the impending death is positive or active euthanasia.

Failure to plug in a respirator, thus permitting natural death to occur, is negative or passive euthanasia.

The public needs to be educated about the implications of both the euthanasia and hospice philosophies. The right-to-live factions oppose not only euthanasia, but they have also begun to oppose hospice, because of misunderstandings of intent. Rather than have the patients prolong their agonizing final days, both programs are channelled to relieve suffering.

The mechanism that might possibly remove this obstacle is legislation, at either the national or state level. As Cicely Saunders wrote of the issue of euthanasia,

> This is an exceedingly difficult and dangerous area in which to introduce legislation. It is difficult because of the inevitable imprecision of key words and the problems of interpretation. Its most dangerous implication is that the incurably ill could all too easily be pressured into feeling that it was their duty to ask for a swift descent into unconsciousness rather than for the attentive concern which may make heavy demands upon those around them.[10]

THE INTERNAL ENVIRONMENT

Not all hospice workers and organizers think that money and material are needed for care of the terminally ill in addition to loving, caring, and psychological support. Altruism is a necessary ingredient, but unlike the hospices of the Middle Ages, the modern hospice cannot exist strictly as an eleemosynary program. Personnel must be paid, and rent, supplies, transportation, and other expenses must be met. If a physical facility is part of the program, then capital funding must be secured. Today, philanthropy has decreased to the point where other sources of operational funding are necessary for the survival of the hospice movement.

All segments of the public must be educated concerning the hospice philosophies. Also included should be hospice workers, organizers, and volunteers, some of whom enter the programs with preconceived ideas and biases that can either slow or hamper development.

The attitude of the hospice workers is crucial. Positive attitudes will result in advancement of the movement, while negative attitudes about what can and should be done for terminally ill patients and their families can only impede progress.

ORGANIZATIONAL STRUCTURE

Though there are several organization models and a number of variations and combinations, we should be alert to the possibility that newer and possibly better structures will surface in the future. We should not be unduly influenced by the few "experts" and their opinions. Hospice developers must keep an open mind to all the existing models and to those that might become available in the future so that they can pick and choose the best features of each for their own particular geographical and environmental needs.

The use of volunteers must be studied in greater detail. Some hospices use either professional or lay volunteers, while others utilize both groups. We may find in the future that different volunteer skills can and should be utilized. If so, hospice developers should not be reluctant to experiment and adapt for the hospice models of the future.

THE TEAM NEED

The interdisciplinary team is a central theme of hospice. At this writing, there are no formal training courses in the United States specifically for hospice caregivers. Therefore, recruitment, selection, training, and integration of all the needed professional disciplines are difficult to achieve. In time, programs will be introduced in medical schools and in schools of nursing, physical therapy, social work, and chaplaincy, all coordinated by professional thanatologists. For the time being, however, the need to develop the necessary skills and to integrate the necessary professionals into a multidisciplinary team is an obstacle not easily overcome by developing hospices. The desire to serve terminally ill patients and their families under the aegis of hospice is essential for each caregiver and is essential to the development of the team.

NOTES

1. "The 'How To' of Hospice Care," Third National Hospice Symposium, Dominican College Campus, San Rafael, California, May 26–28, 1977.
2. Michael Van Scoy-Mosher, in testimony before California Legislature Assembly Committee on Health, Public Hearing on Hospices, Santa Barbara, California, December 1, 1977.
3. Ibid.
4. "The Hospice Movement," Unpublished Management Services Special Report (Newport Beach, California: Advanced Health Systems, Inc., October 1977).
5. William Lamers, Medical Director, Hospice of Marin, in testimony before California Legislature Assembly Committee on Health, loc. cit.

6. Personal letter from Lawrence D. Burke, Program Director for Rehabilitation Treatment, Rehabilitation & Continuing Care Branch (DCCR), HEW, National Cancer Institute, Bethesda, Maryland, December 15, 1977.

7. Hillhaven Hospice, Tucson, Arizona; Hospice, Inc., New Haven, Connecticut; and Riverside Hospice, Boonton Township, New Jersey.

8. Leda R. Judd, "Hospices—A Background Paper," Unpublished report prepared for HEW, n.d., p. 23.

9. Ibid.

10. Cicely Saunders, "Care for the Dying," *Patient Care* 3 (June 1976).

Chapter 13

Prognostication and Recommendations

Better is the end of a thing than the beginning thereof.
Ecclesiastes 7:8

PROGNOSTICATION

What is the future of hospices? This fledgling movement in the United States is likely to expand at a rather rapid rate for the next five to ten years; then, growth will probably level off. A number of opportunists will enter the field hoping to make a quick profit. Some of the better-managed hospital chain companies will explore hospice and will undoubtedly succeed within the free enterprise system. Others, though, the fly-by-nighters, will enter the field, and only through the diligence and perseverance of the conscientious hospice operators will these shady operators be forced to fall by the wayside.

Although, by their very nature, institutional hospices cry out for free-standing facilities to house them, the United States, with its proliferation of general acute hospital beds, will undoubtedly opt for the general hospital models. Alternatively, some nursing homes will be converted for use as free-standing hospices.

Home care will be the most popular hospice model. In order to develop at all, many hospices will have to follow the home care model, beginning with all-volunteer programs, both professional and lay. Gradually, funding will be secured for operating expenses, with volunteers augmented by part-time personnel. Ultimately, most part timers will be replaced by full-time personnel. As funding for each home care hospice becomes more readily available, the hospice will be able to handle progressively more and more patients, to the limit of its resources.

Institutional hospices will combine home care models with their own, either as an adjunct to their own organizations, or under contract with separate home care hospice organizations. Conversely, the home care hospice models will ultimately merge with hospital models, or they will contract separately for inpatient hospice beds; this, for example, is the current arrangement between Hospice of Santa Barbara and Pinecrest Hospital in Santa Barbara, California.

Although at present there is a general unawareness of hospice throughout American society, the public will become gradually aware of hospice over the next two years, after which an information explosion will burst upon the scene. This will thus aid the development of hospices. Awareness will come about because of the educational efforts of medical schools, nursing schools, allied health training programs, practicing hospice practitioners, universities, hospitals, and others interested in hospice education.

Although only a trickle of third-party reimbursement is available today, as more and more states experiment with hospice and subsequently legislate new hospice programs, reimbursement will become more readily available. The next five to ten years are crucial in this regard, but as the public is educated, legislators also will become more knowledgeable and will insist upon reasonable regulatory agency regulations that will promote the hospice idea and permit adequate remuneration for services provided.

RECOMMENDATIONS

- Analysis of the results of the legislation survey showed that the most pressing need is for education of both U.S. and Canadian lawmakers. They need in-depth information about terminal illness and about the change in philosophy from strictly *curing* to *caring,* to palliation when curing is not feasible. Even though many states and some provinces do not have operative hospices, numerous groups are forming in all parts of both countries to learn and teach the hospice philosophy. Lawmakers at both the state and federal levels should avail themselves of these resources. In those states where hospices exist or are forming, legislators can benefit by the experiences of these hospices, by either conducting hearings similar to the December 1, 1977 California Assembly Health Committee hearing previously cited, or by making fact-finding visits to the operational hospices.

- An additional important need is for education of the policy makers of all the nation's insurance companies. They also need in-depth information about terminal illness and about the change in philosophy from curing to caring when curing is not feasible. Insurance coverage for family members and the bereaved is just as important as coverage for the terminally ill patient.

• Similar education of the general public and health professionals is needed. The education process can take place through lectures, seminar workshops, university extension courses, and the like, sponsored by:

1. The National Hospice Organization
2. Regional hospice associations, e.g., the Southern California Hospice Association and the Northern California Component of State Hospice Committee
3. Operational hospices in the United States and palliative care services in Canada
4. Special hospital educational programs
5. University credit and noncredit courses
6. Other national medical, hospital, and allied health organizations, such as the American Medical Association, American Osteopathic Association, American Hospital Association, Federation of American Hospitals, American Public Health Association, American College of Hospital Administrators
7. State, regional, and local medical societies, hospital organizations, mental health organizations, allied health groups, and the like
8. Government agencies at the federal, state, and local levels
9. Community and church groups, discussion groups, clubs, and organizations
10. Television, newspapers, magazines, professional journals, and other media

• The nation's universities, high schools, and grade schools should adopt formal courses covering dying and death. Death education of the future citizens of this country must begin in the primary and secondary schools. Although a few progressive schools have begun sporadic classes, organized programs covering all facets of thanatology are needed in every school in the country. Progressive school administrators are hereby challenged to innovate in their own districts in this vital area of needed education.

• The nation's lawmakers and their advisors in the departments of health at both the state and federal levels need to understand that the care for the terminally ill patients currently provided in most hospitals and nursing homes is not hospice care. Health professionals employed by the states and provinces must be made to understand the total philosophy of hospice care, especially the central theme that the patient *and* the family are the unit care. Only then can these health professionals properly adivse their respective legislative bodies on hospice programs.

- Society has a tremendous need to correct its generally fallacious thinking about euthanasia and the right of the individual to die. Responsive legislation will help in this direction, and the 35 states that have either right-to-die acts or pending bills have made positive first steps. However, only the passage of time, additional enactments, and subsequent amendments will begin the process of correcting this thinking.

- Third-party payers tend to tie their reimbursement policies to state licensure. If this practice prevails, it is incumbent upon lawmakers to classify and license hospice programs properly. On the other hand, if licensure will mean oppressive regulation, then hospice development will be stifled. The question of licensure needs to be debated in open forums by all states' lawmakers.

- Legislators need to understand that hospice is a *program,* not necessarily a *facility*. A home care type of hospice can be just as effective as a free-standing hospice or a hospice that is part of a general acute-care hospital. An understanding of this program-versus-facility distinction is important, because it can channel future legislation into the most productive forms of hospice development; a misunderstanding can stifle growth.

- The lawmakers from the 15 states that have no right-to-die acts or bills must examine the motivations and political machinations and ask if the failure to draft right-to-die legislation will benefit the citizens of their respective states. In recent years, legislation regarding rights of individuals has proliferated. Is not the right-to-die as important as other rights of the individual?

- The legislators in the eight states that have enacted natural death laws must listen to the objections raised by the people of their respective states regarding that legislation. Amendments are needed that will improve the laws and better serve the needs of the people rather than serving only the special interests that have lobbied for specific features.

- Insurance companies need to re-examine their policy of providing benefits only for medical services that treat the condition. Society is now concerned with treating the *patient* when it is no longer desirable to treat the condition. The wholistic approach rather than disease curing must be the new emphasis.

- Insurance companies need to examine their policy of providing benefits only for in-hospital services. Terminally ill patients can be effectively treated at home, in a free-standing hospice facility, or as outpatients. Further studies must, of course, be performed to show that hospice care in these settings is cost-effective.

• The term *custodial care* needs to be disassociated from terminally ill patients. True care of terminally ill patients is not custodial care. A precise definition of terminal illness must be accepted by legislators and insurance companies. Knowledge of hospice care performed will come as a result of education.

• The federal government, under Titles XVIII and XIX of the Social Security Act (Medicare and Medicaid), must recognize the need for cost reimbursement to health professionals who care for terminally ill patients. The old definitions, standards, and philosophies of care for the terminally ill and their families must be revised. A beginning has been made with the definition of hospice adopted by the U.S. Congress (see the glossary), but a planned, overall approach is needed now.

• More research and pilot projects by insurance companies are needed now. All progressive insurance companies should get on the band wagon and perform a needed service to society.

• Insurance companies need to include specific, defined hospice benefits in their policies in order to determine equitable rates actuarially. By refusing to pay benefits because certain services are not currently considered hospital services, insurance companies are doing a disservice to the hospitals, the terminally ill patients and their families, and society at large.

• To prevent abuses of benefits yet to be designed, insurance companies need to establish adequate controls that will ensure insurance beneficiaries and health care providers of their fair shares of the insurance dollar.

• There is a need for a public policy that will recognize that when a person's brain is dead, the entire person is dead, that at this point, there is neither life nor hope, in spite of respiration and heartbeat that are continued by mechanical means.

• More research is needed on health professionals', patients', and others' attitudes towards death. This will help channel care of the terminally ill patients into the most productive and satisfying avenues for both the patients and the providers of care.

• Medical schools need to prepare physicians-in-training in how to deal with death and dying. They need to stress that terminally ill patients require different modalities than do acutely ill patients. Physicians need to learn the difference between the philosophy of curing and the philosophy of caring and palliation when curing is not feasible. Similar training is needed for all other health professionals and nonprofessionals who may be involved in the care of terminally ill patients.

• Many terminally ill patients suffer excruciating pain. Some patients who cannot tolerate morphine or other pain-killing drugs could be successfully treated with heroin, administered in the proper dosages and with the proper frequency. United States lawmakers must be brought to the realization that the legalization of heroin will be a tremendous service to some terminally ill patients. Lawmakers' and physicians' fears that the patients will become addicted to the narcotic are pointless, since these patients generally have only days or weeks of life before them.

• Research studies need to be made to explore the cost of hospice services as compared to the cost of similar services that can be performed in general acute-care hospitals and skilled nursing facilities.

• The states should develop guidelines for the purpose of assuring the public that the highest quality of care will be rendered to the terminally ill. However, restraint should be exercised in promulgating regulations for the control of hospices. Unduly demanding, picayune, and onerous government regulations could have an inhibitory effect on developing hospices instead of encouraging the growth of this infant discipline. State governments should offer assistance rather than take an adversary stance, as in recent years some state departments of health have taken towards hospitals and convalescent homes.

• Additional studies are needed to determine the most efficacious organizational hospice models for varying conditions. For example, is home care or inpatient care most effective for patients with varying diagnoses? Which model is the most cost-effective? Does the age of the patient have a bearing on the cost of providing care? What is the optimum staffing pattern? Should the services provided for patients and families vary according to the relationship and the number of family members? Is there any difference in care of the patients with no family members?

• Studies are needed to project the number of hospice programs needed, by model, in order to design the proper number of patient units and their optimum geographical distribution. Controls need to be considered so that hospices do not proliferate to the detriment of the patient units. We must avoid "too much hospice" if we are to maintain the optimum level of quality of services.

Glossary[1]

Acute Disease. A disease characterized by a single episode of a fairly short duration from which the patient returns to a normal or previous state and level of activity. While acute diseases are frequently distinguished from chronic diseases, there is no standard definition or distinction. It is worth noting that an acute episode of a chronic disease (e.g., an episode of diabetic coma in a patient with diabetes) is often treated as an acute disease.

Admission. The formal acceptance by a hospital or other inpatient health care facility of a patient who is to be provided with room, board, and continuous nursing service in an area of the hospital or in a facility where patients generally stay at least overnight.

Admitting Health Personnel. Specially trained and licensed (when necessary) health workers other than physicians, dentists, podiatrists, and nurses. The term has no constant or agreed-upon detailed meaning; sometimes it is used synonymously with paramedical personnel, sometimes it means all health workers who perform tasks that must otherwise be performed by a physician, and sometimes it refers to health workers who do not usually engage in independent practice.

Admitting Physician. The physician responsible for admission of a patient to a hospital or other inpatient health facility. The physician may remain responsible for the care of the patient once admitted (*see* Private Patient), or not (the housestaff usually becomes responsible). At some facilities, all admitting decisions are made by a single physician called an admitting physician; this is typically a rotating responsibility.

Alternatives to Long-Term Institutional Care. The whole range of health, nutritional, housing, and social services designed to keep people, particularly the aged, disabled, and retarded, out of institutions, such as skilled nursing facilities, that provide care on a long-term basis. The goal is to provide the range of services necessary to allow the person to continue to function in the home. Alternatives to long-term care include day-care centers, foster homes or homemaker services.

Ancillary Services. Hospital or other inpatient health program, services other than room and board, and professional services. They may include x-ray, drug, laboratory, or other services not separately itemized, but the specific content can be quite variable.

Attending Physician. The physician legally responsible for the care given a patient in a hospital or other health program. Usually a private patient's private physician who is also responsible for the patient's outpatient care. The attending physician for a public patient is typically chosen by the hospital, upon the patient's admission, from among members of its medical staff, or is one of its teaching physicians.

Bed. A bed in a hospital or other inpatient health facility. Many definitions require that the beds be maintained for continuous (24-hour) use by inpatients. Beds are often used as a measure of capacity; hospital sizes are compared by comparing their number of beds. Licenses and certificates of need may be granted for specific numbers or types of beds, e.g., surgical, pediatric, obstetric, or extended-care. Facilities may have both licensed and unlicensed beds, and active and licensed but unused beds. Other qualifying adjectives are frequently used to categorize.beds, e.g., available, occupied, acute-care or observation beds.

Beneficiary. A person who is eligible to receive, or is receiving, benefits from an insurance policy (usually) or health maintenance organization (occasionally). Usually includes both people who have themselves contracted for benefits and their eligible dependents.

Benefit. In insurance, a sum of money provided for certain types of loss or for covered services, under the terms of a policy. The benefits may be paid to the insured or to others on the insured's behalf. In prepayment programs such as HMOs, benefits are the services the program will provide a member whenever needed and to the extent needed.

Blue Cross Association (BCA). The national nonprofit organization to which the 70 Blue Cross plans in the United States voluntarily belong. BCA administers programs of licensure and approval for Blue Cross plans, provides specific services related to the writing and administering of health care benefits across the country, and represents the Blue Cross plans in national affairs. Under contract with the Social Security Administration (SSA), BCA is intermediary in the Medicare program for 77 percent of the participating providers (90 percent of the participating hospitals, 50 percent of the participating skilled nursing facilities, and 76 percent of the participating home health agencies).

Blue Cross Plan. A nonprofit, tax-exempt, prepayment health service organization providing coverage for health care and related services. The individual plans should be distinguished from their national association, the Blue Cross Association. The plans were largely the creation of the hospital industry and designed to provide hospitals with a stable source of revenues. Formal association between the Blue Cross and American Hospital Associations ended in 1972. A Blue Cross plan must be a non-profit community service organization whose governing body includes a majority of public representatives. Most plans are regulated by state insurance commissioners under special enabling legislation. Plans are exempt from federal income taxes, and, in most states, from state taxes (both property and premium). Unlike most private insurance companies, the plans usually provide service rather than indemnity benefits and often pay hospitals on the basis of reasonable costs, rather than charges. There are 70 plans in the United States.

Blue Shield Plan. A nonprofit, tax-exempt plan, of a type originally established in 1939, which provides coverage of physicians' services. The individual plans should be distinguished from the National Association of Blue Shield plans. Blue Shield coverage is commonly sold in conjunction with Blue Cross coverage, although this is not always the case. The relationship between Blue Cross and Blue Shield plans has been a cooperative one; it is not uncommon for the two organizations to have a common board and one management and to be located in the same building. Blue Shield's group and individual plans cover some 65 million Americans. In addition, plan activities affect some 20 million people through various government programs, including Medicare (32 plans act as carriers under part B), Medicaid, and CHAMPUS. Most states have enacted special enabling legislation for the Blue plans.

Boarding Homes. Organized or informal facilities that for a fee provide room, board (to those desiring it, often the aged), and, sometimes, custodial care. The provision of medical supervision, social activities, or counseling is not normally included. They are not licensed as health facilities and usually are not subject to licensure at all.

Brain Death. For all legal purposes, a human body with irreversible cessation of total brain function shall, according to usual and customary standards of medical practice, be considered dead.[2]

Carrier. A commercial health insurer, a government agency, or a Blue Cross or Blue Shield plan that underwrites or administers programs that pay for health services. Under the Medicare Part B (Supplemental Medical Insurance) Program and the Federal Employees Health Benefits Program, carriers are agencies and organizations with which the program contracts for administration of various functions, including payment of claims.

Chronic Disease. Diseases that have one or more of the following characteristics: are permanent, leave residual disability, are caused by nonreversible pathological alteration, require special training of the patient for rehabilitation, or may be expected to require a long period of supervision, observation, or care. *See also* Acute Disease.

Clinic. A facility, or part of one, for diagnosis and treatment of outpatients. Clinic is irregularly defined, sometimes either including or excluding physicians' offices, sometimes being limited to facilities that serve poor or public patients, and sometimes being limited to facilities in which graduate or undergraduate medical education takes place.

Custodial Care. Board, room, and other personal assistance services that are generally provided on a long-term basis and that do not include a medical component. Such services are generally not paid for under private or public health insurance or medical care programs, except as incidentals to medical care that a hospital or nursing home inpatient receives. *See also* Boarding Homes.

Death. The cessation of life; ceasing to exist; defined by physicians as a total stoppage of the circulation of the blood, and a cessation of the animal and vital functions consequent thereon, such as respiration, pulsation, etc.[3] *See also* Brain Death.

Disease. Literally, without ease. May be defined as a failure of the adaptive mechanisms of an organism to counteract adequately, normally, or appropriately the stimuli and stresses to which it is subject, resulting in a disturbance in the function or structure of some part of the organism. This definition emphasizes that disease is multifactorial and may be prevented or treated by changing any of the factors. Disease is a very elusive and difficult concept to define, being largely socially defined. Thus, criminality and drug dependence presently tend to be seen as diseases, when they were previously considered moral or legal problems.

Dying. In the case of progressive incurable illness, the last three months of life are generally regarded as the period called "dying." However, it is difficult to determine accurately the duration of life remaining to a person.[4]

Euthanasia. Literally, a good or easy death. Passive euthanasia is desisting from or discontinuing useless prolongation; an act of omission that permits natural death to occur. Active euthanasia may be either indirect or direct. Indirect active euthanasia is indirectly causing death by use of pain-relieving drugs that clearly hasten death. Direct active euthanasia is deliberately inducing death to terminate hopeless suffering or a meaningless existence.[5]

Extended Care Facility (ECF). Previously used in Medicare to mean a skilled nursing facility that qualified for participation in Medicare. In 1972, the law was amended to use the more generic term *skilled nursing facility* for both Medicare and Medicaid. Medicare coverage is limited to 100 days of posthospital extended care services during any spell of illness; thus, Medicare coverage in a skilled nursing facility is limited in duration, must follow a hospital stay, and must be for services related to the cause of the hospital stay. These conditions do not apply to skilled nursing facility benefits under Medicaid. Thus, the term *extended care facility benefits* continues to be used as a kind of shorthand to refer to the benefit limitations on skilled nursing facility care under Medicare.

Extended Care Services. As used in Medicare, services in a skilled nursing facility provided for a limited duration (up to 100 days during the spell of illness) after a hospital stay and for the same condition that caused the hospital stay. As defined under Medicare, the following items and services furnished to an inpatient of a skilled nursing facility are included: nursing care provided or supervised by a registered professional nurse; bed and board associated with the nursing care; physical, occupational, or speech therapy furnished by the skilled nursing facility or by others under arrangements with the facility; medical social services; such drugs, biologicals, supplies, appliances and equipment as are ordinarily used in care and treatment in the skilled nursing facility; medical services provided by an intern or resident of a hospital with which the facility has a transfer agreement; and other services as are necessary to the health of the patients.

Facilities. Buildings, including physical plant, equipment, and supplies, used in providing health services. They are one major type of health resource and include hospitals, nursing homes, and ambulatory care centers, but usually not the offices of individual practitioners.

Full-Time Equivalent Personnel (FTE). Since health care organizations generally employ many part-time personnel for varying schedules in addition to full-time personnel, the number of personnel has little meaning. However, by converting the hours of service to FTE, a meaningful figure can be computed. FTE is found by dividing the total hours of service by the hours usually provided by one full-time person; e.g., 180 total hours of service provided in one week divided by 40 hours per week per full-time person equals 4.5 FTE.[6]

Gork. Originally an acronym for "God only really knows," and then used by housestaff for patients whose problems were so mysterious as to defy diagnosis. It has now lost all connection with its original meaning and is used offensively to describe patients who are, and are likely to remain, comatose.

Health. Defined by the World Health Organization as "a state of complete physical, mental, and social well-being and not merely the absence of disease or infirmity." Experts recognize however, that health has many dimensions (anatomical, physiological, and mental) and is largely culturally defined. The relative importance of various disabilities will differ depending upon the cultural milieu and the role of the affected individual in that culture. Most attempts at measurement have taken a negative approach in that the degree of ill health has been assessed in terms of morbidity and mortality. In general, the detection of changes in health status is easier than the definition and measurement of the absolute level of health.

Health Facilities. Collectively, all buildings and facilities used in the provision of health services. Usually limited to facilities built for the purpose of providing health care, such as hospitals and nursing homes, and, thus, not including an office building in which a physician's office is located. Health facilities, with health personnel, are the principal health resources used in producing health services.

Home Health Agency. An agency that provides home health care. To be certified under Medicare, an agency must provide skilled nursing services and at least one additional therapeutic service (physical, speech, or occupational therapy; medical social services; or home health aide services) in the home.

Home Health Care. Health services rendered to an individual as needed in the home. Such services are provided to aged, disabled, sick, or convalescent people who do not need institutional care. The services may be provided by a visiting nurse association (VNA), home health agency, hospital, or other organized community group. They may be quite specialized or comprehensive (nursing services, speech, physical, occupational, and rehabilitation therapy; homemaker and social services). Under Medicare, such services must be provided by a home health agency. Under Medicaid, states may, but do not have to, restrict coverage of home health care to services provided by home health agencies.

Homemaker Services. Nonmedical support services (e.g., food preparation, bathing) provided to homebound individuals, who are unable to perform these tasks themselves. Such services are not covered under the Medicare and Medicaid programs or most other health insurance programs, but may be included in the social service programs developed by the states under Title XX of the Social Security Act. Homemaker services are intended to preserve independent living and normal family life for the aged, disabled, sick, or convalescent. *See also* Alternatives to Long-Term Institutional Care.

Hospice. A program that provides palliative and supportive care for terminally ill patients and their families, either directly or on a consulting basis with the patient's physician or with another community agency such as a visiting nurse association. Originally a medieval name for a way station where crusaders could be replenished, refreshed, and cared for; used here for an organized program of care for people going through life's last station. The whole family is considered the unit of care, and care extends through the mourning process. Emphasis is placed on symptom control and preparation for, and support before and after, death.

Hospital. An institution whose primary function is to provide inpatient services, diagnostic and therapeutic, for a variety of medical conditions, both surgical and nonsurgical. In addition, most hospitals provide some outpatient services, particularly emergency care. Hospitals are classified by length of stay (short-term or long-term), as teaching or nonteaching, by major type of service (psychiatric, tuberculosis, general, maternity, children's, or ear, nose, and throat), and by control (government, federal, state or local), and as for profit (proprietary) or nonprofit. The hospital system is dominated by the short-term, general, nonprofit community hospital, often called a voluntary hospital.

House Officers. *See* House Staff.

House Staff. Generally, the physician staff in training at a hospital, principally made up of the hospital's interns, residents, and fellows. Members of the house staff are called house officers. Occasionally also applies to physicians salaried by a hospital who are not receiving any graduate medical education.

Illness. Usually used synonymously with disease. Can be differentially defined by saying that illness is present when people perceive themselves as diseased and that disease is present when identifiable by objective, external criteria.

Inpatient. A patient who has been admitted at least overnight to a hospital or other health facility (which is therefore responsible for the patient's room and board) for the purpose of receiving diagnostic, treatment, or other health services. Inpatient care means the care given inpatients.

Insurance. The contractual relationship that exists when one party, for a consideration, agrees to reimburse another for loss to a person or thing caused by designated contingencies. The first party is the insurer; the second, the insured; the contract, the insurance policy; the consideration, the premium; the person or thing, the risk; and the contingency, the hazard or peril. Generally, a formal social device for reducing the risk of losses for individuals by spreading the risk over groups. Insurance characteristically, but not necessarily, involves equitable contributions by the insured, pooling of risks, and the transfer of risks by contract. Insurance may be offered on either a profit or nonprofit basis, to groups or individuals.

Intensive Care Unit (ICU). A specialized nursing unit that concentrates, in one area within a hospital, seriously ill patients needing constant nursing care and observation. Some intensive care units limit their services to certain types of patients such as coronary care, surgical intensive care, and newborn intensive care units.

Intermediary. A public or private agency or organization selected by providers of health care that enters into an agreement with the secretary of HEW under the Hospital Insurance Program (Part A) of Medicare, to pay claims and perform other functions for the secretary with respect to such providers. Usually, but not necessarily, a Blue Cross plan or private insurance company.

Intermediate Care Facility (ICF). An institution recognized under the Medicaid program that is licensed under state law to provide, on a regular basis, health-related care and services to people who do not require the degree of care or treatment that a hospital or skilled nursing facility is designed to provide, but who because of their mental or physical condition require care and services (above the level of room and board) that can be made available to them only through institutional facilities. Public institutions for care of the mentally retarded or people with related conditions are also included. The distinction between health-related care and services and room and board is often difficult to make but is important because ICFs are subject to quite different regulation and coverage than institutions that do not provide health-related care and services. An ICF/MR is an ICF that cares solely or particularly for the mentally retarded.

Length of Stay (LOS). The length of an inpatient's stay in a hospital or other health facility. It is one measure of use of health facilities, reported as an average number of days spent in a facility per admission or discharge. It is calculated as follows: total number of days in the facility for all discharges and deaths occurring during a period divided by the number of discharges and deaths during the same period. Average lengths of stay vary and are measured for people with various ages, specific diagnoses, or sources of payment.

License. A permission granted to a person or organization by competent authority, usually public, to engage in a practice, occupation, or activity otherwise unlawful. Licensure is the process by which the license is granted. Since a license is needed to begin lawful practice, it is usually granted on the basis of examination and/or proof of education rather than measures of performance. When given, licenses are usually permanent but may be conditioned on annual payment of a fee, proof of continuing education, or proof of competence. Common grounds for revocation of a license include incompetence, commission of a crime (whether or not related to the licensed practice), or moral turpitude. Possession of a medical license from one state may or may not suffice to obtain a license from another. There is no national licensure system for health professionals, although requirements are often so nearly standardized as to constitute a national system.

Licensed Practical Nurse (LPN). A nurse who has practical experience in the provision of nursing care but is not a graduate of a formal program of nursing education. The education, required experience, licensure, and job responsibilities of LPNs vary.

Licensed Vocational Nurse (LVN). *See* Licensed Practical Nurse.

Long-Term Care. Long-term health and/or personal care services provided in an institution or at home to people who are chronically ill, aged, disabled, or retarded. The term is often used more narrowly to refer only to long-term institutional care such as that provided in nursing homes, homes for the retarded, and mental hospitals. Ambulatory services, like home health care, which also can be provided on a long-term basis, are seen as alternatives to long-term institutional care.

Major Surgery. Surgery in which the operative procedure is hazardous. Major surgery is irregularly distinguished from minor surgery according to whether or not it requires a general anesthetic, involves an amputation above the ankle or wrist, or includes entering one of the body cavities (abdomen, chest, or head).

Malingering. The willful, deliberate, and fraudulent feigning or exaggeration of the symptoms of illness or injury done for the purpose of a consciously desired end, such as collecting insurance or some other benefit.

Medicaid (Title XIX). A federally aided, state-operated and -administered program that provides medical benefits for certain low-income people in need of health and medical care. The program, authorized by Title XIX of the Social Security Act, is basically for the poor. It does not cover all of the poor, however, but only those who are members of one of the categories of people who can be covered under the welfare cash payment programs: the aged, the blind, the disabled, and members of families with dependent children where one parent is absent, incapacitated, or unemployed. Under certain circumstances, states may provide Medicaid coverage for children under 21 who are not categorically related. Subject to broad federal guidelines, states determine the benefits covered, program eligibility, rates of payment for providers, and methods of administering the program. Medicaid is estimated to provide services to some 25 million people.

Medi-Cal. California's Medicaid program.

Medical Assistance Program. The health care program for the poor authorized by Title XIX of the Social Security Act, known as Medicaid.

Medical Staff. Collectively, the physicians, dentists, and other professionals responsible for medical care in a health facility, typically a hospital. Such staff may be full-time or part-time, employed by the hospital or not, and include all professionals who want to be included (open staff) or just those who meet various standards of competence (closed staff). Staff privileges may or may not be permanent or conditioned on continued evidence of competence.

Medicare (Title XVIII). A nationwide health insurance program for people aged 65 and over, for persons eligible for social security disability payments for over two years, and for certain workers and their dependents who need kidney transplantation or dialysis. Health insurance protection is available to insured people without regard to income. Monies from payroll taxes and premiums from beneficiaries are deposited in special trust funds for use in meeting the expenses incurred by the insured. The program was enacted July 30, 1965 as Title XVIII—Health Insurance for the Aged—of the Social Security Act and became effective on July 1, 1966. It consists of two separate but coordinated programs: hospital insurance (Part A), and supplementary medical insurance (Part B).

Medicine. The art and science of promoting, maintaining, and restoring individual health, and of diagnosing and treating disease.[7]

Minor Surgery. Surgery in which the operative procedure is not hazardous, e.g., repair of lacerations, treatment of fractures, and biopsies. *See also* Major Surgery.

Morbidity. The extent of illness, injury, or disability in a defined population. It is usually expressed in general or specific rates of incidence or prevalence. Sometimes used to refer to any episode of disease. *See also* Mortality.

Mortality. Death. Used to describe the relation of deaths to the population in which they occur. The mortality rate (death rate) expresses the number of deaths in a unit of population within a prescribed time and may be expressed as crude death rates (e.g., total deaths in relation to total population during a year) or as rates specific for diseases and, sometimes, for age, sex, or other attributes (e.g., number of deaths from cancer in white males in relation to the white male population during a year).

Nurse. A person whose primary responsibility is the provision of nursing care. A nurse can be defined as a professional person qualified by education and authorized by law to practice nursing. Not all people who fit the initial definition are nurses (for example, nurses' aides). There are many different types, specialities, and grades of nurses whose titles generally describe their special responsibilities (charge or head, hospital, private or private-duty, public health, and school nurses).

Nursing Care. Care to assist people, sick or well, in the performance of those activities contributing to health or its recovery (or to peaceful death) that they would perform unaided if they had the necessary strength, will, or knowledge. This includes assisting patients in carrying out therapeutic plans initiated by physicians and other health professionals and assisting other members of the medical team in performing the nursing function and understanding patients' health needs. The specific content of nursing care varies in different countries and situations, and it is important to note that, as defined, it is not given solely by nurses but also by many other health workers.

Nursing Homes. Generally, a wide range of institutions, other than hospitals, that provide various levels of maintenance and personal or nursing care to people who are unable to care for themselves and who may have health problems ranging from minimal to very serious. The term includes free-standing institutions or identifiable components of other health facilities that provide nursing care and related services, personal care, and residential care. Nursing homes include skilled nursing facilities, intermediate-care facilities, and extended-care facilities, but not boarding homes.

Occupational Therapist. A specially trained person who evaluates the self-care, work, and leisure performance skills of well and disabled clients of all age ranges and who plans and implements programs and social and interpersonal activities designed to restore, develop, and/or maintain the clients' ability satisfactorily to accomplish those daily living tasks required of their specific ages and necessary to their particular occupational roles. There were 11,200 registered occupational therapists in 1972, an estimated 3,500 of whom were not in practice. About four-fifths of occupational therapists work in hospitals, others are employed in nursing homes and extended or long-term care facilities, rehabilitation centers, schools and camps for handicapped children, community health agencies, and educational and research institutions. Formal educational preparation of an occupational therapist requires at least four academic years of college or university work leading to a baccalaureate degree, plus a minimum of six months' field work experience. Those who already have a baccalaureate degree in a field other than occupational therapy may enroll in a postbaccalaureate program leading to a master's degree in occupational therapy or a certificate of proficiency in occupational therapy.

Outpatient. A patient who is receiving ambulatory care at a hospital or other health facility without being admitted to the facility. Usually does not mean people receiving services from a physician's office or other program that does not also give inpatient care. Outpatient care refers to care given to outpatients, often in organized programs.

Outpatient Medical Facility. A facility designed to provide a limited or full spectrum of health and medical services (including health education and maintenance, preventive services, diagnosis, treatment, and rehabilitation) to individuals who do not require hospitalization or institutionalization.

Paramedical Personnel. Those health personnel who are not doctors. It includes medical technicians, health aides, record keepers, family health workers, nutritionists, dental hygienists, physician assistants, and health associates, but there seems to be no agreed-upon list of included occupations.

Patient. One who is receiving health services; sometimes used synonymously with consumer. *See also* Inpatient, Outpatient, Private Patient, and Service Patient.

Patient Days. A measure of institutional use, usually expressed as the number of inpatients at a specified time (e.g., midnight).

Physical Therapist. A specially trained and licensed individual who uses physical agents, biomechanical and neurophysiological principles, and assistive devices in relieving pain, restoring maximum function, and preventing disability following disease, injury, or loss of a bodily part. The number of people employed as physical therapists reached 16,500 in 1973. It is estimated that approximately 8,000 are employed in hospitals, while others are employed by public health agencies and by rehabilitation centers, schools, or societies for crippled children. A license is required to practice physical therapy in the 50 states, the District of Columbia, Puerto Rico, and the Virgin Islands. To obtain a license, an applicant must have a baccalaureate degree or certificate from an approved school of physical therapy and must pass a state board examination, where required.

Practical Nurse. *See* Licensed Practical Nurse.

Primary Care. Basic or general health care that emphasizes the point when the patient first seeks assistance from the medical care system and the care of the simpler and more common illnesses. The primary care provider usually also assumes ongoing responsibility for the patient in both health maintenance and therapy of illness. Primary care is comprehensive in the sense that it takes responsibility for the overall coordination of the care of the patient's health problems, be they biological, behavioral, or social. The appropriate use of consultants and community resources is an important part of effective primary care. Such care is generally provided by physicians but is increasingly provided by other personnel such as family nurse practitioners.

Private Patient. A patient whose care is the responsibility of an identifiable individual health professional (usually a physician) who is paid directly (by the patient or a third party) for service to the patient. The physician is called a personal physician and the patient is the physician's private patient. Private patients are contrasted with public, service, or ward patients whose care is the responsibility of a health program or institution. Public patients are often cared for by an individual practitioner paid by the program (such as a member of the house staff), but the program, rather than the individual, is paid for the care. The distinction is important to third-party payers (including Medicare) because situations arise in which payment is made to both a program and an individual practitioner for the same services. The term occasionally refers to a patient occupying a private room in an institution.

PRN. Abbreviation for the Latin *pro re nata,* "according as circumstances may require;"[8] as needed.

Provider. An individual or institution that gives medical care. In Medicare, an institutional provider is a hospital, skilled nursing facility, home health agency, or one of certain providers of outpatient physical therapy services. These providers receive cost-related reimbursement. Other Medicare providers, paid on a charge basis, are called suppliers. Individual providers include individuals who practice independently of institutional providers.

Registered Nurse. A nurse who has graduated from a formal program of nursing education and been licensed by appropriate state authority. Registered nurses are the most highly educated of nurses with the widest scope of responsibility, including, at least potentially, all aspects of nursing care.

Registration. The process by which qualified individuals are listed on an official roster maintained by a governmental or nongovernmental agency. Standards for registration may include such things as successful completion of a written examination given by the registry, membership in the professional association maintaining the registry, and education and experience such as graduation from an approved program or equivalent experience. Registration is a form of credentialing, similar to certification. Registration is also used to describe the recording of notifiable diseases, or the listing and follow-up of patients with such diseases.

Secondary Care. Services provided by medical specialists who generally do not have first contact with patients (e.g., cardiologists, urologists, dermatologists). In the United States, however, there has been a trend toward self-referral by patients themselves for these services, rather than referral by primary care providers. This route is quite different from the path usually followed in England, for example, where all patients first seek care from primary care providers and are then referred to secondary and/or tertiary providers, as needed. *See also* Tertiary Care.

Service Patient. A patient whose care is the responsibility of a health program or institution (usually a hospital). Service patients are often cared for by an individual practitioner paid by the program (typically a member of a hospital's house staff), but the program, not the individual, is paid for the care. Sometimes called a public or ward patient. *See also* Private Patient.

Skilled Nursing Facility (SNF). Under Medicare and Medicaid, an institution (or a distinct part of an institution) that has in effect a transfer agreement with one or more participating hospitals and that—

- is primarily engaged in providing skilled nursing care and related services for patients who require medical or nursing care, or rehabilitation services for the rehabilitation of the injured, disabled, or sick;
- has formal policies developed with the advice of a group of professional personnel, including one or more physicians and one or more registered nurses, to govern the skilled nursing care and related medical or other services it provides;
- has a physician, a registered professional nurse, or a medical staff responsible for the execution of such policies; and
- has a requirement that the health care of every patient be under the supervision of a physician and provides for having a physician available to furnish necessary medical care in case of an emergency (and meets other specific requirements of the law).

Social Worker. A professionally trained person providing social services, either as a member of a health team, a social service section of a health facility, or on a consultant basis. Social services are provided to enable a patient, family members, or others to deal with problems of social functioning affecting the health or well-being of the patient. Most trained social workers now hold a master's degree in social work (M.S.W.). A B.A. in social work (B.S.W.) is a beginning professional degree. It is estimated that there are some 120,000 to 140,000 trained social workers in the current social service labor force of about 300,000 social service workers. Approximately 30,000 of that larger number are employed in health-related settings. Social workers increasingly are engaging in private and independent practice, on both a full-time and part-time basis. Eighteen states (including Puerto Rico) now regulate social work, with six licensing independent practice specifically. An estimated 30,000 social workers are engaged in some degree of independent practice. The National Association of Social Workers (NASW) requires that social workers engaging in independent practice have at least an M.S.W. and two years of professionally supervised practice in the methods to be employed in independent practice.

Staff Privilege. Sometimes called admitting, hospital, practice, or clinical privilege. The privilege, granted by a hospital or other inpatient health program, to a physician or other independent practitioner, to join the hospital's medical staff and hospitalize private patients in the hospital. A practitioner is usually granted privileges after meeting certain standards, being accepted by the medical staff and board of trustees of the hospital, and pledging to carry out certain duties for the hospital such as teaching without pay or providing emergency or clinic services. Most community and other private hospitals in this country are staffed by physicians who are private practitioners and obtain access to hospital facilities in this manner. It is common for a physician to have staff privileges at more than one hospital. On the other hand, since hospitals accept only a limited number of physicians, some practitioners are excluded and end up with no access to hospital facilities, having no staff privileges. The standards used to determine staff privileges sometimes include evaluation by the county medical society, which may give preference to or require membership in that society, which may in turn require membership in the American Medical Association. This practice is formally opposed by the AMA. Some hospitals limit privileges for certain services to board-eligible or certified physicians. Full-time, or hospital-based, physicians and physicians working in a system such as a prepaid group practice with its own hospital are not usually thought of as having staff privileges. Many hospitals have several different types of grades of staff privileges with names such as active, associate, courtesy, or limited; however, these names have irregular and unsystemized meaning, although the real differences between the different types of privileges deserve a decent nomenclature.

Standards. Generally, a measure set by competent authority as the rule for measuring quantity or quality. Conformity with standards is usually a condition of licensure, accreditation, or payment for services. Standards may be defined in relation to the actual or predicted effects of care; the performance or credentials of professional personnel; and the physical plant, governance, and administration of facilities and programs.

Terminal Condition. An incurable condition caused by injury, disease, or illness that, regardless of the application of life-sustaining procedures, will, according to reasonable medical judgment, produce death, and where the application of life-sustaining procedures serves only to postpone the moment of the patient's death.[9]

Tertiary Care. Services provided by highly specialized providers such as neurologists, neurosurgeons, thoracic surgeons, and intensive care units. Such services frequently require highly sophisticated technological and support facilities. The development of these services has largely been a function of diagnostic and therapeutic advances attained through basic and clinical biomedical research. *See also* Primary Care and Secondary Care.

Therapy. The treatment of disease.

Third-Party Payer. Any organization, public or private, that pays or insures health or medical expenses on behalf of beneficiaries or recipients (e.g., Blue Cross and Shield, commercial insurance companies, Medicare, and Medicaid). The individual generally pays a premium for such coverage in all private and in some public programs. The organization then pays bills on the individual's behalf; such payments are called third-party payments and are distinguished by the separation between the individual receiving the service (the first party), the individual or institution providing it (the second party), and the organization paying for it (the third party).

Title XVIII. The title of the Social Security Act that contains the principal legislative authority for the Medicare program.

Title XIX. The title of the Social Security Act that contains the principal legislative authority for the Medicaid program.

Treatment. The management and care of a patient for the purpose of combating disease or disorder.

Turkey. Deprecating house staff term for an inpatient whom they feel does not need hospital admission. Such patients are not usually malingerers.

Visit. An encounter between a patient and a health professional that requires the patient to travel from home to the professional's usual place of practice (an office visit), or vice versa (a house call or home visit).

Visiting Nurse Association or **Visiting Nurse Service (VNA).** A voluntary health agency that provides services in the home, including health supervision, education, and counseling; bedside care; and the carrying out of physicians' orders using nurses and other personnel such as home health aides specifically trained for specific tasks of personal bedside care. These agencies had their origin in the 1870s in the visiting or district nursing provided to sick poor in their homes by such voluntary agencies as the New York City Mission. The first visiting nurse associations were established in Buffalo, Boston, and Philadelphia in 1886 and 1887. *See also* Home Health Agency.

NOTES

1. Unless otherwise specified, all terms are as defined in *A Discursive Dictionary of Health Care*, 94th Congress, 2nd Session (Washington, D.C.: U.S. Government Printing Office, 1976).
2. M. DeMere et al., "Report on Definition of Death, from Law and Medicine Committee" (Chicago: American Bar Association, 1975).
3. *Black's Law Dictionary*, 4th ed. (St. Paul: West Publishing Co., 1968), p. 488.
4. Richard Lamerton, *Care of the Dying* (Westport, Connecticut: Technomic Publishing Co., 1976), p. 13.
5. O. Ruth Russell, *Freedom to Die* (New York: Human Sciences Press, 1975), p. 23.
6. The author's definition.
7. *Random House Dictionary of the English Language* (New York: Random House, 1967), p. 1,039.
8. *Dorland's Illustrated Medical Dictionary*, 24th ed. (Philadelphia: W. B. Saunders, 1965), p. 1,218.
9. Section 7187(f) of the California Health and Safety Code.

Appendix A

Listing of Hospices

This appendix is a partial listing of hospices, either operative or in various stages of development. Although some of the organizations listed may not yet be true hospices as defined by the National Hospice Organization (NHO), at the time of this listing preparation they were in process of developing or expanding their services to meet the definition. Identification information has come from numerous sources. Accuracy of information, therefore, cannot be guaranteed. The reader is referred to the NHO for the most current information.

Eastern United States

CONNECTICUT

The Connecticut Hospice, Inc.
Formerly known as Hospice, Inc.
765 Prospect St. (203) 787-5779 Home Care
New Haven, Conn. 06511 (203) 787-5871 General Offices
Dennis Rezendes, Executive Director

DELAWARE

Wilmington Medical Center
501 W. 14th St., Box 1668
Wilmington, Delaware 19889 (302) 428-1212
Bernard Z. Paulshock, M.D.

MAINE

Hospice of Maine, Inc.
32 Thomas St.
Portland, Maine 04122 (207) 774-4417
Rev. S. George Bovill

Clover Manor Hospice
440 Minot Ave.
Auburn, Maine 04210 (207) 784-3575
William Gillis

MARYLAND

Church Hospital Corporation
100 N. Broadway
Baltimore, MD 21231 (301) 732-4730, x 386
Dan W. McAdams, Vice President

Deer's Head Hospital Center
Box 2018
Salisbury, MD 21801 (301) 742-2164
Edward G. Phoebus, JD

Holy Cross Hospital
1500 Forest Glen Rd.
Silver Spring, MD 20910 (301) 565-0100
Peg O. McCuiston

MASSACHUSETTS

Hospice of the Good Shepherd
1671 Beacon St.
Waban, MA 02168 (617) 244-4028
Philip Kelleher

Rose Hawthorne Lathrop Home
Woodman & Bay Streets
Fall River, MA 02724

University of Massachusetts Medical Center
55 Lake Ave., N.
Worcester, MA 01605 (617) 856-2233
Dr. Melvin Krant

Youville Rehabilitation & Chronic Disease Hospital
1575 Cambridge St.
Cambridge, MA 02138 (617) 876-4344
Sister Annette Caron, Executive Director

NEW HAMPSHIRE

Salemhaven, Inc.
8 Pleasant St.
Salem, New Hampshire 03079
Rev. Daniel V. Weaver, Vice President

NEW JERSEY

Beth Israel Hospital
70 Parker Ave.
Passaic, N.J. 07055
Judy Iverson, R.N., Department Head,
Tri-Hospital Home Care Project

Hospice-Overlook Home Care
52 North Hillside Ave.
Chatham, N.J. 07928
Denis Manger, R.N.

Hunterdon Medical Center
Flemington, N.J. 08822
Linda A. McGreevy, R.N., Supervisor Home Care

Newark Beth Israel Medical Center
201 Lyons Ave.
Newark, N.J. 07112
Mrs. Miriam Hirsch

Overlook Hospital
193 Morris Ave.
Summit, N.J. 07901 (201) 522-2114
L. Stephen Hartford, Vice President—Ambulatory Services

Riverside Hospice
c/o Riverside Hospital
Boonton Township, N.J. 07005 (201) 335-6121
Donald Wernsing, M.D., Medical Director
Mrs. Carol Dayton, Project Director

NEW YORK

Burke Rehabilitation Center
785 Mamaroneck Ave.
White Plains, N.Y. 10605 (914) 948-0050 x 2270
Fletcher McDowell, M.D., Medical Director
Charlotte M. Hamill, Associate Director

Calvary Hospital
1600 Macombs Rd.
Bronx, N.Y. 10452 (212) 299-7800
Lorraine Tregde, President - Executive Director
Ronald Lavalle, Administrator

Capitol District Hospice, Inc.
1166 Avon Rd.
Schenectady, N.Y. 12308 (418) 374-2201
Catherine Woodford

Haven of Schenectady
2217 Niskayuna Drive
Schenectady, N.Y. 12309
Mrs. Jeanette Neisuler

Hospice Buffalo, Inc.
2929 Main St.
Buffalo, N.Y. 14214 (716) 838-4438
Charlotte Shedd, Chairman of the Board

Hospice Committee
RD 2, Box 96
Corning, N.Y. 14830
Mrs. Nina McPhilmy, Chairman

Hospice Oneida
95 Genesee St.
Clinton, N.Y. 13323
Patricia Meyer, c/o Dr. William Krause

Hospice of Putnam County, Inc.
Glen Ridge Road
Mahopac, N.Y. 10541 (914) 628-5917
Maralyn Carr

Hospice of Rockland, Inc.
4 Union Road
Spring Valley, N.Y 10977
Joe Brass, Executive Director
Dr. Alan J. Tuckman

Hospice of Westchester
35 Apawamis Ave.
Rye, N.Y. 10580 (914) 967-3840
Charlotte M. Duncan

Isabella Geriatric Center
New York, N.Y. 10040
Florence Safford, D.S.W.

Our Lady of Lourdes Memorial Hospital
169 Riverside Drive
Binghamton, N.Y. 13905
David M. Bloom, M.D., Vice President for Medical Affairs

Roosevelt Hospital
Advanced Disease Service
428 West 59th St.
New York, N.Y. 10019
William Fisher, M.D.

Rosary Hill Home
600 Linda Ave.
Hawthorne, N.Y. 10532

St. Joseph's Hospital and Nursing Home
127 South Broadway
Yonkers, N.Y. 10701 (914) 965-6700
Sr. Frances Mallon

St. Luke's Hospital Center
114th St. & Amsterdam Ave. (212) 870-1732 or
New York, N.Y. 10025 (212) 870-6775
Gary Gambuti, Executive Vice President
Chaplain Carleton Sweetser, Chairman Hospice Committee

St. Vincent's Hospital and Medical Center of New York
153 West 11th St.
New York, N.Y. 10011 (212) 790-7508
Sr. Ellen Burke

St. Rose's Home
71 Jackson
New York, N.Y. 10001

Syosset Hospital
225 Jericho Turnpike
Syosset, N.Y. 11791 (516) 921-7000
Richard W. Hahn, Administrator

University of Rochester Cancer Center
Box 704
601 Elmwood Ave.
Rochester, N.Y. 14642

NORTH CAROLINA

Glenn R. Frye Memorial Hospital
420 North Center St.
Hickory, N.C. 28601 (704) 322-6070
Ann H. Thomas, R.N.

Hospice at Charlotte, Inc.
Professional Services Center
403 N. Tryon St. - Suite 304
Charlotte, N.C. 28202 (704) 375-0100
Zach Thomas III

Hospice of Gastonia, NC, Inc.
Box 3535, Akers Station
Gastonia, N.C. 28052 (704) 864-7201
Rev. Robert E. Johnson

Hospice of North Carolina, Inc.
Box 11452
Winston-Salem, N.C. 27106 (919) 724-7122
Peter Keese, President
Carl Whitney, Executive Director

Hospice of Winston-Salem/
Forsyth County, Inc.
Forsyth Memorial Hospital
333 Silas Creek Parkway
Winston-Salem, N.C. 27103 (919) 768-3972
George W. Bowman III

Lower Cape Fear Hospice
c/o Wilmington Health Associates
1202 Medical Center Dr.
Wilmington, N.C. 28401
Daniel Gottovi, M.D.

Mountain Area Hospice
P.O. Box 8404
Asheville, N.C. 28804 (704) 252-7138
Rev. Richard C. Swogger

Sandhills Area Hospice
Moore Memorial Hospital
P.O. Box 3000
Pinehurst, N.C. 28374 (919) 295-1000
Chaplain M. Carlisle Franks

Triangle Hospice
P.O. Box 3120
Chapel Hill, N.C. 27514 (919) 929-1020
Vivian Dixon

PENNSYLVANIA

Butterfly Hill-Hospice for Children
4401 Pine St.
Philadelphia, PA 91904
Rev. Dan Sullivan, Chairperson
Ms. Heidi Wells, Secretary, Board of Directors

Forbes Health System-Hospice
500 Finley St.
Pittsburgh, PA 15206 (412) 665-3533
Rose Ferraro

Harrisburg Hospital Hospice Unit
S. Front St.
Harrisburg, PA 17101 (717) 652-3000
Joyce Ukema, R.N.

Hospice Inc. of Greene County
Greene County Memorial Hospital
Bonar Ave.
Waynesburg, PA 15370 (412) 627-3101
Barbara DeHaas

Lutheran Welfare Service of
N.E. Pennsylvania
143 W. Broad St.
Hazleton, PA 18201 (717) 455-7578
Rev. John M. Brndjar

Paoli Memorial Hospital
Lancaster Pike
Paoli, PA 19301 (215) 648-1206
Wm. Michael Tomlinson

Sacred Health Home
1315 West Hunting Park Ave.
Philadelphia, PA 19133

St. Christopher's Hospital for Children
2600 N. Lawrence St.
Philadelphia, PA 19133

RHODE ISLAND

Hospice Care of Rhode Island, Inc.
1085 N. Main St.
Warwick, R.I. 02904 (401) 274-8941
Robert J. Canny

VERMONT

Task Force for Hospice of
Vermont Ecumenical Council
P.O. Box 593
Burlington, VT (802) 862-8498
Ann M. Jarvey

VIRGINIA

Haven of Northern Virginia
7300 McWhorter Pl.
Annandale, VA 22003 (703) 941-7000
Dorothy N. Garrett, Coordinator

The Hospice of Loudon, Prince
William & Western Fairfax Counties, Inc.
1633 Washington Plaza
Reston, VA 22090 (703) 437-5100
Barbara D. Webster

Riverside Hospital
500 J. Clyde Morris Blvd.
Newport News, VA 23601 (804) 599-2020
Gerald R. Brink

St. Mary's Hospital
5801 Bremo Rd.
Richmond, VA 23226 (804) 285-2011
Katherine Webb, MSW, Hospice Planner

WASHINGTON, D.C.

Georgetown University Hospital
3800 Reservoir Rd., N.W.
Washington, D.C. 20007
Josefina Magno, M.D., Director Medical Oncology
Charles M. O'Brien, Administrator

Washington Hospice Society, Inc.
1511 K St., N.W.
Washington, D.C. 20005 (202) 638-1300
Sister Mary Margaret Meldon, Executive Director

Midwestern United States

ILLINOIS

Chicago Hospice, Inc.
10630 Torrance Ave.
Chicago, IL 60617 (312) 721-2061

Evangelical Hospital Association (UCC)
1415 W. 22nd St.
Oak Brook, IL 60521 (312) 986-6399
Larry K. Ulrich

Highland Park Hospital
718 Glenview Ave.
Highland Park, IL 60035 (312) 432-8000
Marge Lyons, R.N., Counselor

Horizon Hospice
2430 N. Lakeview
Chicago, IL 60614 (312) 327-8086
Ada Addington

Hospice of the North Shore
c/o North Shore Senior Center
Rm. 106, Winnetka Community House
620 Lincoln
Winnetka, IL 60093 (312) 446-8750

Lutheran General Hospital
Cancer Care Center
1775 Dempster St.
Park Ridge, IL 60068
Robert Lehner, Unit Administrator

St. Barnabas Hospice
672 Riford Rd.
Glen Ellyn, IL 60137
Clarice A. D'Addio

St. John's Hospital
Southern Illinois University School of Medicine
Department of Family Practice
P.O. Box 3926
Springfield, IL 62708 (217) 782-5872
James Cox, M.D.

INDIANA

Hospice of Fort Wayne Inc.
c/o Allen County Cancer Society
2925 East State St.
Fort Wayne, IN 46805 (219) 432-3615
Sherri Jackson, Coordinator

Hospice of St. Joseph County
c/o Dr. Gerhart Niemeyer
806 E. Angela Blvd.
South Bend, IN 46617 (219) 234-9949
Dr. Gerhart Niemeyer

Methodist Hospital of Indiana, Inc., Hospice Unit
1604 N. Capitol Ave.
Indianapolis, IN 46260 (317) 924-8794
Dr. William Elliott, Chairman Hospice Task Force

Parkview Hospice
2200 Randalia Dr.
Fort Wayne, IN 46805 (219) 484-6636
Donald K. Reeves

IOWA

Drake University
Des Moines, IA 50322
Dr. W. D. Blanks, Professor of Religion

Hospice of Central Iowa, Inc.
635 - 46th St.
Des Moines, Iowa 50312 (515) 279-5403

KENTUCKY

Community Hospice
Ephraim McDowell Community Cancer Network
915 South Limestone
Lexington, KY 40503 (606) 233-6541

Hospice of Louisville and Southern Indiana
233 E. Grey St., Suite 602
Louisville, KY 40202 (502) 584-4834
A. Robert Crawford, Jr.

MICHIGAN

Hospice of Flint, Inc.
G-2474 S. Ballenger Rd.
Flint, MI 48507 (313) 232-4023
Bruce Marshall

Hospices of Michigan
Grace Hospital, Room 407
4160 John Rd.
Detroit, MI 48201
Dr. William L. Simpson, President

Hospice of Greater Grand Rapids
Emeritus Center - Aquinas College
Grand Rapids, MI 49506 (616) 774-1233
Kent M. Batley

St. Joseph Mercy Hospital
P.O. Box 995
Ann Arbor, MI 48106
Helen V. Berg

MINNESOTA

Bethesda Lutheran Hospice
Bethesda Lutheran Hospital
559 Capitol Rd.
St. Paul, MN 55103 (612) 221-2298 or 2376
Dr. Robert S. Brown, Medical Director
Carmian M. Seifert, R.N., MPH, Associate Director

Coalition for Terminal Care
University YMCA
1425 University Ave., SE
Minneapolis, MN 55414 (612) 373-9700

Fairview Community Hospitals
2312 South 6th St.
Minneapolis, MN 55406 (612) 371-6300
C. N. Platau, President
Dr. Gus Nelson, Hospice Consultant

Our Lady of Good Counsel
2076 St. Anthony Ave.
St. Paul, MN 55104
Sister M. Peter, Administrator

Riveredge Hospice
415 Oak St.
P.O. Box 313
Breckenridge, MN 56520
Sr. Mary Camillus Weier

Saint Joseph's Hospital
69 W. Exchange St.
St. Paul, MN 55102 (612) 291-3122
Gerard W. Frawley

MISSOURI

Hospice Care of Mid America
Truman Medical Center
2301 Holmes St.
Kansas City, MO 64108 (816) 556-3398
Harry Kuba, President
Rev. Carl F. Petering, Vice President

Hospice of Central Missouri
c/o Missouri Cancer Programs
115 Bus Loop 70 West
Columbia, MO 65201 (314) 449-3945 (R. Sonneman)
John H. Walters, M.D.

Lutheran Medical Center, Continuing Care Unit
2639 Miami St.
St. Louis, MO 63118 (314) 772-1456
Robert Kraetsch, M.D., Medical Coordinator
Ruth Reko, Unit Coordinator

Terminal Care Resource Team
800 Stadium Dr.
VA Hospital
Columbia, MO 65201 (314) 443-2511
Chaplain Jay L. Ketchie

OHIO

Barnesville Hospital Assoc., Inc.
639 W. Main St.
Barnesville, OH 43713 (614) 425-3941
Mary DeNoble, R.N., MS

Cancer Center, Inc.
Northeast Ohio Cancer Program
11001 Cedar Ave.
Cleveland, OH 44106 (216) 421-7300
Abraham Brickner, ACSW

Community Home Health Services
2615 East High St.
Springfield, OH 45501 (514) 325-0531 x 318
Joanne W. Smith

Holy Family Home
6707 State Rd.
Parma, OH 44134

Hospice of Cincinnati
P.O. Box 19221
Cincinnati, OH 45219 (513) 721-1444
Ms. Kim Devore

Hospice of Dayton
Room 430
122 East Apple St.
Dayton, OH 45409 (513) 223-0759
Betty L. Schmoll, R.N., MS

Hospice Unit
St. Joseph Hospital
205 W. 20th St.
Loraine, OH 44052 (216) 245-6851
Ronald Streem

Interim Hospice Directional
Committee of Columbus
245 N. Powell Ave.
Columbus, OH 43204
Judith A. Patton

Northwest Ohio Hospice Organization
c/o M.C.O. Cancer Program
C.C. 10008
Toledo, OH 43699 (419) 381-3717
Janet L. Blaufuss

Serene
Cleveland Metropolitan General Hospital
3395 Scranton Rd.
Cleveland, OH 44109

Visiting Nurse Service of Summit County, Inc.
1200 McArthur Dr.
Akron, OH 44320 (216) 745-1601
Joan L. Andrews, R.N.

OKLAHOMA

Tulsa Psychiatric Center
1620 East 12th St.
Tulsa, OK 74120

Peggy Roggenbuck

TENNESSEE

Fort Sanders Presbyterian Hospital Hospice
1909 Clinch Ave., S.W.
Knoxville, TN 37916 (615) 546-2811

Thomas W. Newland, President

WISCONSIN

Bellin Hospice
Bellin Memorial Hospital
744 S. Webster Ave., P.O. Box 1700
Greenbay, WI 54305 (414) 468-3480

Thomas R. Leicht, M.D., Medical Director
Chaplain John Machek
Kathryn Andrews, R.N.

Hospice of Milwaukee
1035 Alfred St.
Brookfield, WI 53005 (414) 272-3028

Rev. Michael Stoltman

Milwaukee Hospice, Inc.
3402 W. State St.
Milwaukee, WI 53208 (414) 271-3686

Rev. Jim Evans

Rogers Memorial Hospital
34810 Pabst Rd.
Oconomowoc, WI 53066 (414) 567-5535, 367-3172

Rev. Michael J. Stolpman, Acting Director
Caryl A. Huige, Administrative Assistant

Sacred Heart Hospital
900 W. Clairmont Ave.
Eau Claire, WI 54701

Sister Augusta Sperl

Southern United States

ALABAMA

The Hospice of Mobile, Inc.
409 Pine Court
Mobile, AL 36608 (205) 473-4423
Ed Lakeman

ARKANSAS

Hospice of Arkansas, Inc.
2200 Hidden Valley Dr.
Little Rock, AR 72212 (501) 224-4858
Ms. B. J. Chick

FLORIDA

Elisabeth Kubler-Ross Hospice, Inc.
P.O. Box 6311
Clearwater, FL 33518 (813) 461-5125
Leo Gamow, Interim Administrative Director

Hospice of Miami
127 N.E. 4 Street
Miami, FL 33132 (305) 371-0927
High Westbrook

Hospice Orlando
P.O. Box 8581
Orlando, FL 32806 (305) 647-2523
Daniel C. Hadlock, M.D., Medical Director
Lynn Hadlock, Patient Care Coordinator

Hospice of Palm Beach County, Inc.
P.O. Box 6562
W. Palm Beach, FL 33405 (305) 582-0143
Stella Monchick, R.N., B.H.S.

Hospice of St. Francis, Inc.
P.O. Box 5563
Titusville, FL 32780 (305) 267-2842
Emilie Sasko, R.N.

GEORGIA

Hospice Atlanta, Inc.
1055 McLynn Ave., N.E.
Atlanta, GA 30306 (404) 875-6963
Harry Hamil, Coordinator of Board of Directors

Our Lady of Perpetual Help Hospital
760 Washington St., S.W.
Atlanta, GA 30315

Wesley Homes, Inc.
1817 Clifton Rd., N.E.
Atlanta, GA 30329 (404) 325-2988
T. Scott Harstan

TEXAS

Home Health-Home Care, Inc.
904 N. 28th St.
Orange, TX 77630 (713) 886-0141
Louise Jones Maberry

Hospice of North Texas, Inc.
P.O. Box 2028
Dallas, TX 75220 (214) 422-2730
James J. Spencer, Executive Director

Southeast Texas Hospice
312 Pine St.
Orange, TX 77630 (713) 886-0622
Judge Homer E. Stephenson, President of Board
Joan Lyons, Secretary of Board

Western United States

ARIZONA

Hillhaven Hospice
5504 E. Pima
Tucson, AZ 85712 (602) 886-8263
Sister Teresa Marie McIntier, Executive Director

Hospice of the Valley
P.O. Box 5436
908 N. 24th St.
Phoenix, AZ 85008 (602) 273-1978
Sister Evangela Hanfland

Life Service Center
3550 North Central Ave., Suite 324
Phoenix, AZ 85012
Sharol Cannon, Director

Valley of the Sun Hospice
3535 E. Lincoln Dr.
Scottsdale, AZ 85253
Rev. Gerald Rosenberry, Director

CALIFORNIA

Ad Hoc Hospice Committee
720 Plymouth Rd.
Claremont, CA 91711 (714) 626-4690
Rev. Worth George, Executive Director of Pilgrim Place
Rev. John W. Flucke

David M. Brotman Hospital, Oncology Unit
3828 Delmas Terrace
Culver City, CA 90230 (213) 836-7000, x 181
Damon DeCrow, Hospital Administrator
Barbara Ruben, MA, Clinical Thanatologist

Camarillo Hospice
P.O. Box 293
Camarillo, CA 93010 (805) 482-8859
Jim Jeffers

Center for Living with the Dying
1500 N. Los Padres Blvd.
Santa Clara, CA (415) 253-0700
Ms. Mary Lynn Swanson

College Park Hospital
6666 Montezuma Rd.
San Diego, CA 92115 (714) 463-8811
S. Saunders, Administrator

Community Support Group-Hospice Concept
21 Willow Rd.
Menlo Park, CA 94025 (415) 321-6691
Joan Parker, Secretary

El Cajon Valley Hospital
1688 E. Main St.
El Cajon, CA 92021 (714) 440-1122
Donald F. Zuercher, Administrator
Jeanne Dennis, MSW

El Camino Hospital, H.E.A.R.T.
2500 Grant Rd., Human Support Office, ECH
Mountain View, CA 94042 (415) 968-8111, x. 44601
R. Edwin Hawkins, Hospital Administrator
Daniel Dugan, Human Support Coordinator

Encino Hospital Palliative Service
16237 Ventura Blvd.
Encino, CA 91316 (213) 986-4500
John Franks, Administrator
Jerry Coash, Director Social & Life Crisis Services

Episcopal Community Services Hospice Group
601 Market St.
San Diego, CA 92101
Charles M. Brown, Staff Associate - Hospice Group

Home Health & Counseling Services, Inc.
110 Petticoat Lane
Walnut Creek, CA 94509 (415) 937-8311
Leonard J. Dolton

Home Hospice of Sonoma County
P.O. Box 3642
Santa Rosa, CA 95402 (707) 542-5045
Lois Simpson, President
Mary L. Barnhisel, Treasurer

Hospice Care Study Group
Community Services Planning Council, Inc.
Upstairs at 1832 Tribute Road
Sacramento, CA 95815 (916) 929-6802
Margaret Fenelon

Hospice of the Conejo
100 E. Thousand Oaks Blvd.
Suite 224D
Thousand Oaks, CA 91360 (805) 495-7464 (On TLC) or 495-2145
Donna Hochberg, Counselor

Hospice of Contra Costa
120 La Case Via
Walnut Creek, CA 94596 (415) 934-5380
Tighe O'Hanrahan

Hospice in the Home
14401 Gilmore St.
Van Nuys, CA 91401

Hospice of Humboldt
c/o St. Luke's Manor Convalescent Hospital
2400 Newburg Rd.
Fortuna, CA 95540 (707) 725-4467
Margaret A. Soderberg, R.N., Director Nursing Services

Hospice Los Angeles
510 Doheny Rd.
Beverly Hills, CA 90210 (213) 397-2379
Lee Goodman-Malamuth, President

Hospice of Marin
P.O. Box 72
Kentfield, CA 94904 (415) 472-7490
William M. Lamers, M.D., Medical Director
Mary Taverna, Executive Director

Hospice of the Monterey Peninsula
P.O. Box 7236
Carmel, CA 93921 (408) 625-0666
Stephen Connor, Executive Director

Hospice of Ojai
22 Taormina Lane
Ojai, CA 93023 (805) 646-5842 or 646-1000
Bernice Small, Coordinator

Hospice Orange County, Inc.
25255 Cabot Rd., Suite 203
Laguna Hills, CA 92653 (714) 837-6500
Jim Jett, M.D., Medical Director
Leo J. Steady, Ph.D., Administrator

Hospice of San Francisco
c/o San Francisco Home Health Service
2940 Sixteenth St., Suite 301
San Francisco, CA 94103 (415) 864-6470
Joyce A. Tufts, Associate Director

Hospice of San Luis Obispo County
257 First St.
Avila Beach, CA 93424
Benjamin Shapiro, President

Hospice of Santa Barbara, Inc.
330 E. Carrillo St.
Santa Barbara, CA 93101 (805) 965-2850
Sidney J. Smith, Executive Director
Valerie Buckley, Office Manager

Hospice of Santa Cruz County
330 Doris Ave.
Aptos, CA 95003 (408) 688-1286
Julie Martin-Pitts

Hospice of Pasadena, Inc.
c/o H. Rex Green, M.D.
960 E. Green St., Suite 209
Pasadena, CA 91106 (213) 796-4337/681-8323

Hospice of Solano
P.O. Box 4442
Vallejo, CA 94590 (707) 553-1322
Bob Noonan, Executive Secretary
Guy W. Grenny, Ph.D., Social Services Chairman

Hospice of Tulare County
226 S. Blackstone
Tulare, CA 93274 (209) 686-8651 or 686-3702
c/o Esther Greenberg, Chairperson

Hospital/Home Health Care
23228 Hawthorne Blvd.
Torrance, CA 90505 (213) 373-6373
Elinor Griffin

In-Home Care System
1870 El Camino Real - Suite 101
Burlingame, CA 94010 (415) 692-0827
Lynette Harris

Inland Hospice Association
600 Avery Rd.
Claremont, CA 91711

Kaiser-Permanente Hayward Hospice
27400 Hesperian Blvd.
Hayward, CA 94545
Norman T. Walter, M.D., Medical Director

Kaiser-Permanente Hospice Program
12500 South Hoxie Ave.
Norwalk, CA 90650 (213) 920-4525
George G. Espe, M.D., Medical Director

Long Beach Community Hospital
1720 Termino Ave.
Long Beach, CA 90801 (213) 597-6655
Bruce Sanderson, Administrator

Mercy Hospice
Clairmont Heights Rd.
Reading, CA 96001 (916) 243-2121, x 413
Dr. John Clark

Mid Peninsula Health Service, Inc.
510 Emerson St.
Palo Alto, CA 94301 (415) 324-1964
Deborah Ridley, R.N., PHN, Home Care Coordinator

Monterey Hospice
Carmel Hill Professional Center
632 Van Buren
Monterey, CA 93940 (908) 373-7275
Dr. Jerry Rubin

National In-Home Health Services
6850 Van Nuys Blvd., Suite 218
Van Nuys, CA 91405 (213) 988-7575
Paul Jarrett, President
Pat Weihe, R.N., Director Nursing Services

O'Connor Hospital
Hospice-Special Support Unit
2105 Forest Ave.
San Jose, CA 95128 (408) 298-3900, x 311
Judith Urrea, Ph.D.

Parkwood Community Hospital
7022 Shoup Ave.
Canoga Park, CA 91304 (213) 348-0500
Charlene Wilson, R.N., Hospice Coordinator

Pinecrest Hospital
2415 De La Vina St.
Santa Barbara, CA 93105 (805) 682-2511, x 142
William F. Maertz, Administrator
Janet Bauer, R.N., Coordinator

Restorative Home Care
3772 Katella Ave.
Los Alamitos, CA 90720 (714) 821-9081 or (213) 598-9756
Judy Ballentine, R.N., Liaison Nurse

St. Agnes Hospital
1303 E. Herndon
Fresno, CA 93710 (209) 431-5000
Sister M. Gladys Marie, CSC, Executive Administrator
Joan Christenson, Administrative Assistant

St. John's Hospital—Mercy Hospice
333 North F Street
Oxnard, CA 93030 (805) 483-1141, x 2175
Richard Towell, Hospital Administrator
Richard Ames, MSW, Director Social Service

San Diego County Hospice Corp.
233 "A" St. - Suite 1212
San Diego, CA 92101 (714) 231-2660
Stephen M. Harmon, Executive Director

San Francisco Regional Cancer Foundation
14th Ave. & Lake St.
San Francisco, CA 94118 (415) 221-2132
John F. O'Brien, Program Administrator

San Pedro & Peninsula Hospital
1300 W. Seventh St.
San Pedro, CA 90732 (213) 547-1146
Mary Dete, R.N., Coordinator

Sequoia Hospital District
Patient Support Program
Whipple & The Alameda
Redwood City, CA 94062 (415) 369-5811, x 693
Dolores Crom

Shanti Project
106 Evergreen Lane
Berkeley, CA 94705 (415) 849-0336
Charles A. Garfield, Ph.D., Director
Rachel Clark, Administrator

Visiting Nurse Association of Los Angeles, Inc.
2530 W. Eighth St.
Los Angeles, CA 90057 (213) 380-3965
Lillian H. O'Brien, R.N., MPH, Executive Director

Visiting Nurse Association, Inc.
5232 Claremont
Oakland, CA 94618 (415) 654-8093
Jane Matkovich, R.N., M.S., Assistant Director

Visiting Nurse Association, Inc., Santa Clara
2216 The Alameda
Santa Clara, CA 95050 (408) 244-1280
Miss Dorothy Krueger, R.N., M.S.

Wadsworth Veterans Administration Medical Center
Palliative Treatment Program (Hospice)
Wilshire and Sawtelle Blvds.
Los Angeles, CA 90073 (213) 824-3138
Edwin J. Olsen, M.D., Medical Director (691/11H)

West Hills Hospital, Oncology Unit
7300 Medical Center Drive
Canoga Park, CA 91307 (213) 884-7060
Richard M. Mastaler, Hospital Administrator
G. Davidson, M.D./B. Zeitz, M.D., Medical Directors
Sondra Daughety, R.N., Oncology Supervisor

COLORADO

Boulder Hospice, Inc.
2118 14th St.
Boulder, CO 80302 (303) 449-7740
J. Beau Bohart, Ph.D., Executive Director

Denver Hospice, Inc.
1551 South Flamingo Way
Denver, CO 80222
Carolyn Jaffee

Georgian House Hospice for Continuing Care
1625 Carr St.
Lakewood, CO 80215 (303) 238-0531
Fr. Paul Von Lobkowitz, O.S.J.

Hospice of Metro Denver
1719 E. 19th Ave., Rm. 256
Denver, CO 80218 (303) 839-6256
Betty L. Gordon, R.N.

Larimer Weld Hospice
2115 51st Ave.
Greely, CO 80631
Hope Cassidy

Penrose Hospital
2215 North Cascade Ave.
Colorado Springs, CO 80907
Sister Myra James, R.N., Administrator
c/o Mrs. James V. Carris
1334 Culebra Ave.
Colorado Springs, CO 80907 (303) 475-2600

HAWAII

St. Francis Hospital
2230 Liliha St.
Honolulu, Hawaii 96817
Sister Maureen Keleher
Rev. Richard L. Frank, O.S.C.

NEVADA

Clark County Health District
625 Shadow Lane
P.O. Box 4426
Las Vegas, NV 89106 (702) 385-1291, x 301
Otto H. Ravenholt, M.D.

Memorial Hospice
Sunrise Hospital
3186 Maryland Parkway
Las Vegas, NV 89109 (702) 731-8000
Ernest Lipman, Assistant Administrator

NEW MEXICO

Hospital Home Health Care
(Hospice Unit)
500 Walter, NE-Suite 316
Albuquerque, NM 87102 (505) 842-5967
Judy Walden, R.N.

OREGON

Hospice of Oregon
P.O. Box 14444
Portland, OR 97214 (503) 625-7329
Joseph J. Adams

Oregon Comprehensive Cancer Program
Task Force on Hospice
Gaines Hall
3181 S.W. Sam Jackson Park Rd.
Portland, OR 97201 (503) 225-8706
Gary A. Jacobsen, M.D.

UTAH

Hospice of Salt Lake
P.O. Box 8631
Salt Lake City, UT 84108 (801) 261-3033
Victoria E. Slater, Executive Director

WASHINGTON

Capitol Hospice of Thurston County
3710 Country Club Dr., NW
Olympia, WA 98502 (206) 866-3700
Cathy Anderson

Hospice of Clallam County
938 Marine Dr.
Port Angeles, WA 98362 (206) 457-7018
Marge Koch

Hospice of Jefferson County
1127 Adams
Port Townsend, WA 98368 (206) 385-4314
Ginger Barrett

Hospice Maranatha
P.O. Box 1724
Spokane, WA 99210 (509) 325-2536
Johnny Cox, R.N., Ph.D.

Hospice of Seattle, Inc.
331 16th Ave., E.
Seattle, WA 98112 (206) 322-1881
Patsy Carter, President, Board of Trustees

Hospice of Snohomish County
1019 Pacific Ave.
Everett, WA 98201 (206) 258-7123
Sr. Georgette Bayless

Hospice of Tacoma
7539 Hegra Rd.
Tacoma, WA 98465 (206) 383-4153
Anne M. Katterhagen, R.N., BSN, Administrator

Hospice of Vancouver
13105 N.W. 36th Ave. (203) 693-7142
Vancouver, WA 98665 c/o Helen M. Donovan R.N.
Marie D. Morrison, R.N., G.N.P., President

Lower Valley Hospice
10th and Tacoma
P.O. Box 663
Sunnyside, WA 98944 (509) 837-2101 x 275
Mike Cunningham

St. Joseph's Hospital
3201 Ellis St.
Bellingham, WA 98225 (206) 734-5400 x 407
Sr. Brigid Collins

Canada

BRITISH COLUMBIA

Vancouver General Hospital
Vancouver, British Columbia
Dorothy Babcock, Administration

MANITOBA

St. Boniface General Hospital Palliative Care Unit
409 Tache Ave.
Winnipeg, Manitoba R2H 2A6
Dr. Paul Henteleff, Director Palliative & Supportive Care Service
Dr. David Skelton, Medical Director

NEWFOUNDLAND

St. Clare's Mercy Hospital
St. John's, Newfoundland A1C 5B8 (709) 579-5031
Sister Mary Fabian

NOVA SCOTIA

Victoria General Hospital
Halifax, Nova Scotia
Norma Wylie, RN

ONTARIO

Grace Hospital
Toronto, Ontario
Major Ruth Walker, Administrator

Hotel Dieu Hospital
Kingston, Ontario
Palliative Care Service Director

Princess Margaret Hospital
Toronto, Ontario
Dr. Ruth Allison

St. Michael's Hospital
30 Bond Street
Toronto, Ontario M5B 1W8 (416) 360-4000
Joan Foy, RN, Head Nurse Palliative Care Programme
Sister Mary Zimmerman, Administrator
Sister Irene McDonald, Asst. Administrator—Patient Care

St. Vincent de Paul Hospital
Brockville, Ontario
Dr. Penelope Brook-Williams

Thames Valley Regional Health Center
London, Ontario
Address to: Mrs. Helen Young
1101 the Parkway
London, Ontario

QUEBEC

Notre Dame Hospital
Montreal, Quebec
Margaret Farley, Social Worker

Royal Victoria Hospital
Palliative Care Service
687 Pine Ave., W.
Montreal, Quebec H3A 1A1
Dr. Balfour Mount, F.R.C.S., Director

British Isles

Birchlands Jewish Hospital
London, England

Copper Cliff Hospice
Brighton, England

Countess Mountbatten House
Moor Green
Southampton, England

Cynthia Spencer House
Northampton, England

Douglas MacMillan Home
North Staffordshire, England

Douglas MacMillan Hospice
Stoke on Trent, England

Douglas MacMillan Unit
King Edward VII Hospital
Midhurst, England

MacMillan Unit
Christchurch, England

Hereford Lodge
London, England

Hostel of God
c/o The Anglican Sisters of St. Margaret
East Grinstead, England

Marie Curie Memorial Foundation
(12 Homes throughout British Isles)

Michael Sobell House
(National Society for Cancer Relief)
30 Dorset Square
London NW1 6QL, England 01-402 8125

Michael Sobell House
Mount Vernon
Northwood, England

New Addenbrooks Hospital
Cambridge, England

Priscilla Bacon Lodge
Colman's Hospital
Norwich, England

Roxburghe House
Tor-Na-Dee Hospital
Aberdeen, Scotland

Roxburghe House
Royal Victoria Hospital
Dundee, Scotland

St. Ann's Hospice
Manchester, England

St. Anne's Hospice
Little Hulton, England

St. Barnabas' Hospice
Worthing, England

St. Catherine's Hospice
Bath, England

St. Christopher's Hospice
51-53 Lawrie Park Road
Sydenham SE 26 6DZ, England 01-778 9252
Dr. Cicely Saunders, O.B.E., Medical Director

St. Columbia's Hospice
Edinburgh, Scotland

St. Joseph's Hospice
Mare Street
Hackney, London E8 4SA, England
Dr. Richard Lamerton

St. Joseph's Hospice
Thornton, England

St. Luke's Nursing Home (Hospice)
Little Common Lane off Abbey Lane
Sheffield, S119HE, England

St. Margaret's Hospice
Clydebank, England

St. Mary's Hospice
Birmingham, England

Sir Charles Hayward House
Sherwood Hospital
Nottingham, England

Sir Michael Sobell House
The Churchill Hospital
Headington, Oxford, England Oxford 64841
R. G. Twycross, MA DM MRCP, Consultant Physician

Tarner Home
Brighton, England

Appendix B
Organizations

This appendix is a partial alphabetical listing of organizations that deal with various aspects of death education, grief, bereavement, euthanasia, hospice, and related issues. For more information on any of these organizations, contact them directly.

American Cancer Society, Inc.
777 Third Avenue
New York, New York 10017

A voluntary organization of about 2.3 million Americans united to conquer cancer through balanced programs of research, education, and patient service and rehabilitation. It has an extensive public education program designed specifically to save more of the 100,000 plus individuals who die of cancer each year because known life-saving steps are not taken in time. Its professional education programs are important adjuncts to the medical, dental, and allied health fields.

The Center for Death Education and Research
1167 Social Science Building
University of Minnesota
Minneapolis, Minnesota 55455

The primary concern of the center is the issues and problems surrounding mortality in contemporary society. The center sponsors research on grief and bereavement and studies of attitudes and responses to death and dying. It serves as the repository for relevant materials and as a focal point for the collection and dissemination of information to professionals as well as the lay public. The center provides speakers to concerned groups and conducts symposia and workshops of interest to the various care-giving professions. Numerous publications are available for purchase.

Concern for Dying (formerly The Euthanasia Educational Council)
250 West 57th Street
New York, New York, 10019

This nonprofit organization is dedicated to promoting the creation of "an environment in which each individual can participate fully in decisions regarding his or her treatment during terminal illness." The organization is based on the belief that society should indicate convincingly that physicians are expected to demonstrate humanistic concerns as well as apply skillful medical practices, that life-support systems should not be used to sustain life in cases of intractable pain or irreversible brain damage, and that medication should be given to dying patients in quantities sufficient to eliminate pain even if it shortens life. The organization sponsors conferences, workshops, and symposia to promote open discussion of death and dying, and it distributes materials related to euthanasia.

The Forum for Death Education and Counseling, Inc.
P.O. Box 1226
Arlington, Virginia 22210

This nonprofit corporation promotes death education and counseling and attempts to upgrade the quality of counseling in the areas of death, dying, and bereavement. It prepares and distributes educational materials and provides periodic conferences and meetings on these topics.

Foundation of Thanatology
630 West 168 Street
New York, New York 10032

This public, tax-exempt, educational and scientific organization is devoted to scientific and humanistic inquiries as well as to the application of knowledge to the subjects of the psychological aspects of dying, reactions to death, loss and grief, and recovery from bereavement. Numerous symposia and an extensive thanatological library are sponsored by the foundation.

Make Today Count
c/o Orville Kelly
P.O. Box 303
Burlington, Iowa 52601

This membership organization with 110 chapters internationally offers guidance and mutual support, promotes openness and honesty, and improves the quality of life for people with life-threatening illnesses and for family members and professionals working with these people. Membership in a local chapter also includes a monthly newsletter of information helpful in reaching the groups' goals.

National Committee on the Treatment of Intractable Pain
c/o Judith H. Quattlebaum, President
P.O. Box 34571
Washington, D.C. 20034

The major purpose of the committee is to promote education and research on more effective management and alleviation of intractable pain—particularly that which is beyond the control of available drugs and conventional techniques. The committee is especially directing its efforts to the legalization of heroin for medical purposes of alleviating pain associated with life-threatening illnesses. They endorse the hospice concepts of care for patients with terminal illnesses.

National Hospice Organization
Dennis Rezendes, Executive Secretary
1750 Old Meadow Road
McLean, Virginia 22101

The goals of this relatively new organization are the design of national standards for hospice care, the accumulation of a common data base of pertinent statistics, and the development of a nationwide information program to inform and educate the public. The organization is about to spearhead a national effort to seek maximum reimbursement from public and private insurors for the cost of hospice care.

National Sudden Infant Death Syndrome Foundation (SIDS)
310 South Michigan Ave.
Chicago, Illinois 60604

This foundation is dedicated to supporting medical research into the cause and prevention of SIDS, helping parents of SIDS infants understand what is known about this mysterious disease so that they may not feel unwarranted guilt over the death of their child, training health professionals to assist SIDS families in their time of loss, and educating the public and the professional community so that misunderstanding of SIDS may be eradicated.

Parents Without Partners, Inc.
7910 Woodmont Avenue
Washington, D.C. 20014

Although this membership organization with chapters across the United States was organized to assist single parents (widowed, divorced, separated, or never married), they especially help widowed parents and their children to cope with grief and bereavement. The organization's purposes are basically educational; they sponsor lectures, discussions, publications, and recreational activities to help the single parent cope with the many problems of a single-parent home.

St. Francis Burial Society
3421 Center Street, N.W.
Washington, D.C. 20010

This organization offers alternatives to those who prefer to minimize the material emphasis of the funeral process. The society provides a quarterly publication and consultation services to its members. It offers a line of wooden coffins, ash boxes, palls, and prayer desks that can be ordered either in kit form or already assembled. The quarterly publication offers information on funeral customs, preplanning funerals, the grief process, theological views of death, and bibliographies.

Shanti Nilaya
P.O. Box 2396
Escondido, California 92025

The fulfillment of a dream of Elisabeth Kubler-Ross, Shanti Nilaya, "a healing and growth center," is the first of a number of such healing centers to be established in other states. The organization helps people to take a positive approach to life and to employ their potential, positive energy for purposeful and creative living. The staff concentrates on caring for the dying and their families and on counseling the handicapped of all ages in coming to grips with their "little deaths."

Society of the Compassionate Friends
U.S. National Headquarters
P.O. Box 3247
Hialeah, Florida 33013

An international organization of bereaved parents who, by having been through their own months or years of heartbreak and social isolation, can help to "assist the relief and alleviation of mental and physical illness, suffering and infirmity among bereaved parents." There are no religious affiliations or dues.

Society for the Right To Die
250 West 57th Street
New York, New York 10019

This organization's purpose is to promote appropriate legislation against "the futile prolongation of the dying process." It publishes a periodically updated legislative manual detailing right-to-die laws and discussing pending legislation.

The Thanatology Librarian
Highly Specialized Promotions
P.O. Box 989
Brooklyn, New York 11202

This subscription service provides news of books on death, bereavement, loss, grief, and related topics. It has a rather extensive bibliography and has developed the Thanatology Book Club.

Widow-to-Widow
Widow's Consultation Center
136 East 57th Street
New York, New York 10022

Primarily an informational and counseling support organization for widows and widowers.

Appendix C

Letter of Transmittal: Insurance Company Survey

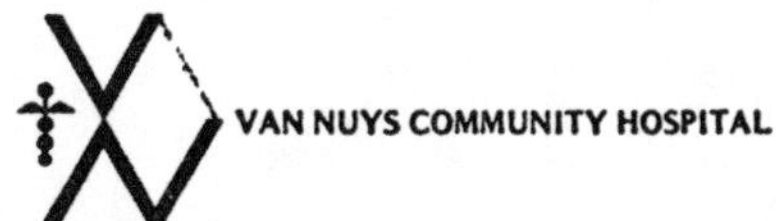

14433 Emelita Street • Van Nuys, California 91401 • Phone [213] 787-1511

October 11, 1977

Gentlemen:

For two reasons I am interested in gathering certain information relating to hospices (see postscript for definition): (1) this hospital is considering the possibility of developing a hospice program, and (2) I am currently preparing a doctoral dissertation entitled "A Study of the Hospice Movement in the United States and Canada". For both purposes the matter of third party payment for hospice services is of great importance.

In order to gather specific information relative to your company's payment practices for hospice services enclosed please find a questionnaire which I would appreciate greatly if you would complete and return in the self-addressed, stamped envelope. The entire questionnaire will take about three minutes to complete, but the results will be of great value to this hospital and to me, personally. The information will be held strictly in confidence, and the results will be tabulated in summary form with no specific identification of any insurance company.

Thank you for your patience and your cooperation. If you are interested in the results of this survey, please check the box in question 11.

Cordially,

Kenneth P. Cohen
Administrator
KPC/br

P.S. Definition of Hospice: A program which provides palliative and supportive care for terminally ill patients and their families, either directly or on a consulting basis with the patient's physician or another community agency such as a visiting nurse association. Originally a medieval name for a way station for pilgrims and travelers where they could be replenished, refreshed, and cared for; used here for an organized program of care for people going through life's last station. The whole family is considered the unit of care and care extends through the mourning process. Emphasis is placed on symptom control and preparation for and support before and after death, full scope health services being provided by an organized interdisciplinary team available on a twenty-four hours-a-day, seven-days-a-week basis.*

* U.S. Congress, House, Committee on Interstate and Foreign Commerce, Sub-Committee on Health and the Environment, A Discursive Dictionary of Health Care, February 1976, 94th Congress, 2nd Session.

Appendix D

Questionnaire: Insurance Company Survey

INSURANCE COMPANY SURVEY

Name of Insurance Company ______________________
Address ______________________
City ______________________ State __________ Zip ________

1. Does your company represent fleet or group of insurance companies? Yes ( ) No ( )
   If yes, how many insurance companies does it represent? __________

2. Is your company or are any companies in the fleet a Medicare Fiscal Intermediary?
   Yes ( ) No ( ) Uncertain ( )

3. Do any of your A & H Plans, group or individual, provide hospice benefits in the following form? (Check all that apply.)
   a) As separate hospice facility ( )
   b) As separate department of general hospital ( )
   c) As home care hospice services ( )
   d) A multidisciplinary team which provides services wherever patient is located in the hospital ( )
   e) Outpatient clinic hospice services ( )
   f) Other. Please specify ______________________ ( )
   ____
   g) None of the above ( )

4. If you provide hospice benefits, what limitations, if any, do your plans impose?
   ____
   ____

5. If you do not provide hospice benefits, are you considering providing in the future?
   Yes ( ) No (

6. If no, and it could be demonstrated that hospice care would be less costly than acute general hospital care, would your company consider paying specific hospice benefits? Yes ( ) No ( ) Uncertain ( )

7. If any of your companies are a Medicare Fiscal Intermediary, do they pay benefits for hospice services? Yes ( ) No ( ) Uncertain ( ) Other ( ), Please specify ______________________

8. Comments or suggestions: ______________________
   ____
   ____

9. Optional: Your Name ______________________ Title __________

10. Department, Division, Etc. ______________________ Date __________

11. If you want to receive a copy of results of this questionnaire, check here ( )

Thank you for your cooperation. You have been of tremendous assistance.

Kenneth P. Cohen, Administrator
Van Nuys Community Hospital
14433 Emelita Street
Van Nuys, California 91401

Appendix E

California Natural Death Act: Guidelines and Directive

These guidelines have been drafted by an ad hoc committee convened at the request of Assemblyman Barry Keene, composed of the Los Angeles County Bar Association's Committee on Bioethics, California Hospital Association Legal Counsel, California Medical Association Legal Counsel and representatives of the Office of Assemblyman Keene.

GUIDELINES FOR SIGNERS

The DIRECTIVE allows you to instruct your doctor not to use artificial methods to extend the natural process of dying.

Before signing the DIRECTIVE, you may ask advice from anyone you wish, but you do not have to see a lawyer or have the DIRECTIVE certified by a notary public.

If you sign the DIRECTIVE, talk it over with your doctor and ask that it be made part of your medical record.

The DIRECTIVE must be WITNESSED by two adults who (1) are not related to you by blood or marriage, (2) are not mentioned in your will, and (3) would have no claim on your estate.

The DIRECTIVE may NOT be witnessed by your doctor or by anyone working for your doctor. If you are in a HOSPITAL at the time you sign the DIRECTIVE, none of its employees may be a witness. If you are in a SKILLED NURSING FACILITY, one of your two witnesses MUST be a "patient advocate" or "ombudsman" designated by the State Department of Aging.

You may sign a DIRECTIVE TO PHYSICIANS if you are at least 18 years old and of sound mind, acting of your own free will in the presence of two qualified witnesses.

No one may force you to sign the DIRECTIVE. No one may deny you insurance or health care services because you have chosen **not** to sign it. If you **do** sign the DIRECTIVE, it will not affect your insurance or any other rights you may have to accept or reject medical treatment.

Your doctor is bound by the DIRECTIVE only (1) if he/she is satisfied that your DIRECTIVE is valid, (2) if another doctor has certified your condition as terminal, and (3) at least 14 days have gone by since you were informed of your condition.

If you sign a DIRECTIVE while in good health, your doctor may respect your wishes but is not bound by the DIRECTIVE.

The DIRECTIVE is valid for a period of five years, at which time you may sign a new one.

The DIRECTIVE is not valid during pregnancy.

You may revoke the DIRECTIVE at any time, even in the final stages of a terminal illness, by (1) destroying it, (2) signing and dating a written statement, or (3) by informing your doctor. No matter how you revoke the DIRECTIVE, be sure your doctor is told of your decision.

Directive to Physicians

Directive made this ______ day of ______________________________ (month, year).

I ______________________________, being of sound mind, willfully, and voluntarily make known my desire that my life shall not be artificially prolonged under the circumstances set forth below, do hereby declare:

1. If at any time I should have an incurable injury, disease, or illness certified to be a terminal condition by two physicians, and where the application of life-sustaining procedures would serve only to artificially prolong the moment of my death and where my physician determines that my death is imminent whether or not life-sustaining procedures are utilized, I direct that such procedures be withheld or withdrawn, and that I be permitted to die naturally.

2. In the absence of my ability to give directions regarding the use of such life-sustaining procedures, it is my intention that this directive shall be honored by my family and physician(s) as the final expression of my legal right to refuse medical or surgical treatment and accept the consequences from such refusal.

3. If I have been diagnosed as pregnant and that diagnosis is known to my physician, this directive shall have no force or effect during the course of my pregnancy.

4. I have been diagnosed and notified at least 14 days ago as having a terminal condition by ______________________________, M.D., whose address is ______________________________ ______________________________, and whose telephone number is ____________________. I understand that if I have not filled in the physician's name and address, it shall be presumed that I did not have a terminal condition when I made out this directive.

5. This directive shall have no force or effect five years from the date filled in above.

6. I understand the full import of this directive and I am emotionally and mentally competent to make this directive.

Signed ______________________________

City, County and State of Residence ______________________________

____

The declarant has been personally known to me and I believe him or her to be of sound mind.

Witness ______________________________

Witness ______________________________

This Directive complies in form with the "Natural Death Act" California Health and Safety Code, Section 7188, Assembly Bill 3060 (Keene).

Summary and Guidelines for Physicians

INTRODUCTION

A person who is at least 18 years of age and of sound mind may sign a DIRECTIVE TO PHYSICIANS as contained in the 1976 California "Natural Death Act." This Act permits a person who meets certain qualifications to give legal effect to his/her wishes to avoid artificial prolongation of the dying process. It also imposes certain obligations—and provides certain protections—for a physician dealing with a person presenting a DIRECTIVE.

SIGNATURE AND WITNESSES

To be effective, the DIRECTIVE must be signed by the patient and witnessed by two persons who are not related to the patient by blood or marriage, are not mentioned in his/her will, are not potential claimants to his/her estate, and are not involved in the patient's medical care. Thus, the DIRECTIVE cannot be witnessed by you or any of your employees. Likewise it should not be witnessed by any other physician or his/her employees, or the employees of any health facility. In addition, if the patient is in a skilled nursing facility at the time of signing, a "patient advocate" or "ombudsman" (designated by the State Department of Aging) must be a witness.

The DIRECTIVE is effective for five years after which a person may sign a new one. A person signing a DIRECTIVE should, if possible, present the document to his/her physician so that it can be made part of his/her current medical record.

EFFECT OF A DIRECTIVE

Upon receipt of a DIRECTIVE from any patient (qualified or unqualified) the attending physician must determine that the DIRECTIVE meets legal requirements. Under the Act a "qualified patient" is a person diagnosed and certified in writing to be afflicted with a terminal condition by two physicians, one of whom shall be the attending physician, who have personally examined the patient.

Whether or not a DIRECTIVE is binding depends upon the condition of the patient at the time the DIRECTIVE was signed.

In order for the DIRECTIVE to be binding the patient must be qualified and have signed or re-executed the DIRECTIVE at least 14 days after being notified of his/her terminal condition. If you do not wish to carry out the DIRECTIVE of such a patient, you are required to transfer care of the patient to a physician who is willing to comply with the DIRECTIVE. If you do not transfer such a patient, you may be found guilty of unprofessional conduct. If you do carry out the DIRECTIVE, you are protected from civil and criminal liability.

The DIRECTIVE is not binding if the patient executed the DIRECTIVE while in good health (in anticipation of a terminal illness or injury). However, should the patient be subsequently diagnosed and certified as terminal, you may carry out the DIRECTIVE if, in your judgment, all of the circumstances known to you justify doing so. If you carry out the DIRECTIVE you are protected from civil and criminal liability.

Regardless of the binding or nonbinding nature of the DIRECTIVE, it is not to be given effect until you have determined that death is imminent, whether or not "life-sustaining procedures" are utilized. Such procedures include mechanical or other "artificial means" which sustain vital functions only to postpone the moment of death. These do not include medications or procedures deemed necessary to alleviate pain.

The DIRECTIVE is invalid and has **no effect** *if the patient is pregnant at the time it is to be carried out.*

REVOCATION

A patient may revoke the DIRECTIVE at any time by (1) destroying it, (2) signing a written statement or (3) communicating to the attending physician his/her wish to revoke the DIRECTIVE. Should you receive such revocation from or on behalf of a patient who has previously signed a DIRECTIVE, enter that information promptly and prominently in the patient's current medical record.

OTHER RIGHTS

No person may be forced to sign a DIRECTIVE. A person who has not signed a DIRECTIVE may not be denied health care or health insurance. The DIRECTIVE has no effect on any insurance policy and does not limit a person's right to accept or reject health care of any kind.

PRECAUTIONS

A person who knowingly conceals or destroys a valid DIRECTIVE is guilty of a misdemeanor. A person who forges or falsifies a DIRECTIVE, or who withholds knowledge of a revocation of a DIRECTIVE may be guilty of unlawful homicide.

SUMMARY

Withholding "life-sustaining procedures" in compliance with a DIRECTIVE is **not** euthanasia or "mercy killing." The DIRECTIVE is **not** a "Living Will." The DIRECTIVE is merely a method, recognized under California law, by which a physician may respect a patient's instruction to permit an imminent death to proceed naturally.

Appendix F

California Natural Death Act

Assembly Bill No. 3060

CHAPTER 1439

An act to add Chapter 3.9 (commencing with Section 7185) to Part 1 of Division 7 of the Health and Safety Code, relating to medical care.

[Approved by Governor September 30, 1976. Filed with Secretary of State September 30, 1976.]

LEGISLATIVE COUNSEL'S DIGEST

AB 3060, Keene. Cessation of medical care for terminal patients.

No existing statute prescribes a procedure whereby a person may provide in advance for the withholding or withdrawal of medical care in the event the person should suffer a terminal illness or mortal injury.

This bill would expressly authorize the withholding or withdrawal of life-sustaining procedures, as defined, from adult patients afflicted with a terminal condition, as defined, where the patient has executed a directive in the form and manner prescribed by the bill. Such a directive would generally be effective for 5 years from the date of execution unless sooner revoked in a specified manner. This bill would relieve physicians, licensed health professionals acting under the direction of a physician, and health facilities from civil liability, and would relieve physicians and licensed health professionals acting under the direction of a physician from criminal prosecution or charges of unprofessional conduct, for withholding or withdrawing life-sustaining procedures in accordance with the provisions of the bill.

The bill would provide that such a withholding or withdrawal of life-sustaining procedures shall not constitute a suicide nor impair or invalidate life insurance, and the bill would specify that the making of such a directive shall not restrict, inhibit, or impair the sale, procurement, or issuance of life insurance or modify existing life insurance. The bill would provide that health insurance carriers, as prescribed, could not require execution of a directive as a condition for being insured for, or receiving, health care services.

The bill would make it a misdemeanor to willfully conceal, cancel, deface, obliterate, or damage the directive of another without the declarant's consent. Any person, not justified or excused by law, who falsifies or forges the directive of another or willfully conceals or withholds personal knowledge of a prescribed revocation with the intent to cause a withholding or withdrawal of life-sustaining procedures contrary to the wishes of the declarant and thereby causes life-sustaining procedures to be withheld or withdrawn, and death to thereby be hastened, would be subject to prosecution for unlawful homicide.

This bill would also provide that, notwithstanding Section 2231 of the Revenue and Taxation Code, there shall be no reimbursement nor appropriation made by this bill for a specified reason.

The people of the State of California do enact as follows:

SECTION 1. Chapter 3.9 (commencing with Section 7185) is added to Part 1 of Division 7 of the Health and Safety Code, to read:

CHAPTER 3.9. NATURAL DEATH ACT

7185. This act shall be known and may be cited as the Natural Death Act.

7186. The Legislature finds that adult persons have the fundamental right to control the decisions relating to the rendering of their own medical care, including the decision to have life-sustaining procedures withheld or withdrawn in instances of a terminal condition.

The Legislature further finds that modern medical technology has made possible the artificial prolongation of human life beyond natural limits.

The Legislature further finds that, in the interest of protecting individual autonomy, such prolongation of life for persons with a terminal condition may cause loss of patient dignity and unnecessary pain and suffering, while providing nothing medically necessary or beneficial to the patient.

The Legislature further finds that there exists considerable uncertainty in the medical and legal professions as to the legality of terminating the use or application of life-sustaining procedures where the patient has voluntarily and in sound mind evidenced a desire that such procedures be withheld or withdrawn.

In recognition of the dignity and privacy which patients have a right to expect, the Legislature hereby declares that the laws of the

State of California shall recognize the right of an adult person to make a written directive instructing his physician to withhold or withdraw life-sustaining procedures in the event of a terminal condition.

7187. The following definitions shall govern the construction of this chapter:

(a) "Attending physician" means the physician selected by, or assigned to, the patient who has primary responsibility for the treatment and care of the patient.

(b) "Directive" means a written document voluntarily executed by the declarant in accordance with the requirements of Section 7188. The directive, or a copy of the directive, shall be made part of the patient's medical records.

(c) "Life-sustaining procedure" means any medical procedure or intervention which utilizes mechanical or other artificial means to sustain, restore, or supplant a vital function, which, when applied to a qualified patient, would serve only to artificially prolong the moment of death and where, in the judgment of the attending physician, death is imminent whether or not such procedures are utilized. "Life-sustaining procedure" shall not include the administration of medication or the performance of any medical procedure deemed necessary to alleviate pain.

(d) "Physician" means a physician and surgeon licensed by the Board of Medical Quality Assurance or the Board of Osteopathic Examiners.

(e) "Qualified patient" means a patient diagnosed and certified in writing to be afflicted with a terminal condition by two physicians, one of whom shall be the attending physician, who have personally examined the patient.

(f) "Terminal condition" means an incurable condition caused by injury, disease, or illness, which, regardless of the application of life-sustaining procedures, would, within reasonable medical judgment, produce death, and where the application of life-sustaining procedures serve only to postpone the moment of death of the patient.

7188. Any adult person may execute a directive directing the withholding or withdrawal of life-sustaining procedures in a terminal condition. The directive shall be signed by the declarant in the presence of two witnesses not related to the declarant by blood or marriage and who would not be entitled to any portion of the estate of the declarant upon his decease under any will of the declarant or codicil thereto then existing or, at the time of the directive, by operation of law then existing. In addition, a witness to a directive shall not be the attending physician, an employee of the attending physician or a health facility in which the declarant is a patient, or any person who has a claim against any portion of the estate of the declarant upon his decease at the time of the execution of the directive. The directive shall be in the following form:

DIRECTIVE TO PHYSICIANS

Directive made this ______ day of ______ (month, year).

I ______, being of sound mind, willfully, and voluntarily make known my desire that my life shall not be artificially prolonged under the circumstances set forth below, do hereby declare:

1. If at any time I should have an incurable injury, disease, or illness certified to be a terminal condition by two physicians, and where the application of life-sustaining procedures would serve only to artificially prolong the moment of my death and where my physician determines that my death is imminent whether or not life-sustaining procedures are utilized, I direct that such procedures be withheld or withdrawn, and that I be permitted to die naturally.

2. In the absence of my ability to give directions regarding the use of such life-sustaining procedures, it is my intention that this directive shall be honored by my family and physician (s) as the final expression of my legal right to refuse medical or surgical treatment and accept the consequences from such refusal.

3. If I have been diagnosed as pregnant and that diagnosis is known to my physician, this directive shall have no force or effect during the course of my pregnancy.

4. I have been diagnosed and notified at least 14 days ago as having a terminal condition by ______, M.D., whose address is ______, and whose telephone number is ______. I understand that if I have not filled in the physician's name and address, it shall be presumed that I did not have a terminal condition when I made out this directive.

5. This directive shall have no force or effect five years from the date filled in above.

6. I understand the full import of this directive and I am emotionally and mentally competent to make this directive.

Signed ______________

City, County and State of Residence ______________

The declarant has been personally known to me and I believe him or her to be of sound mind.

Witness ______________

Witness ______________

7188.5. A directive shall have no force or effect if the declarant is a patient in a skilled nursing facility as defined in subdivision (c) of Section,1250 at the time the directive is executed unless one of the two witnesses to the directive is a patient advocate or ombudsman as may be designated by the State Department of Aging for this purpose pursuant to any other applicable provision of law. The patient advocate or ombudsman shall have the same qualifications as a witness under Section 7188.

The intent of this section is to recognize that some patients in skilled nursing facilities may be so insulated from a voluntary decisionmaking role, by virtue of the custodial nature of their care, as to require special assurance that they are capable of willfully and voluntarily executing a directive.

7189. (a) A directive may be revoked at any time by the declarant, without regard to his mental state or competency, by any of the following methods:

(1) By being canceled, defaced, obliterated, or burnt, torn, or otherwise destroyed by the declarant or by some person in his presence and by his direction.

(2) By a written revocation of the declarant expressing his intent to revoke, signed and dated by the declarant. Such revocation shall become effective only upon communication to the attending physician by the declarant or by a person acting on behalf of the declarant. The attending physician shall record in the patient's medical record the time and date when he received notification of the written revocation.

(3) By a verbal expression by the declarant of his intent to revoke the directive. Such revocation shall become effective only upon communication to the attending physician by the declarant or by a person acting on behalf of the declarant. The attending physician shall record in the patient's medical record the time, date, and place of the revocation and the time, date, and place, if different, of when he received notification of the revocation.

(b) There shall be no criminal or civil liability on the part of any person for failure to act upon a revocation made pursuant to this section unless that person has actual knowledge of the revocation.

7189.5. A directive shall be effective for five years from the date of execution thereof unless sooner revoked in a manner prescribed in Section 7189. Nothing in this chapter shall be construed to prevent a declarant from reexecuting a directive at any time in accordance with the formalities of Section 7188, including reexecution subsequent to a diagnosis of a terminal condition. If the declarant has executed more than one directive, such time shall be determined from the date of execution of the last directive known to the attending physician. If the declarant becomes comatose or is rendered incapable of communicating with the attending physician, the directive shall remain in effect for the duration of the comatose condition or until such time as the declarant's condition renders him or her able to communicate with the attending physician.

7190. No physician or health facility which, acting in accordance with the requirements of this chapter, causes the withholding or withdrawal of life-sustaining procedures from a qualified patient, shall be subject to civil liability therefrom. No licensed health professional, acting under the direction of a physician, who participates in the withholding or withdrawal of life-sustaining procedures in accordance with the provisions of this chapter shall be subject to any civil liability. No physician, or licensed health professional acting under the direction of a physician, who participates in the withholding or withdrawal of life-sustaining procedures in accordance with the provisions of this chapter shall be guilty of any criminal act or of unprofessional conduct.

7191. (a) Prior to effecting a withholding or withdrawal of life-sustaining procedures from a qualified patient pursuant to the directive, the attending physician shall determine that the directive complies with Section 7188, and, if the patient is mentally competent, that the directive and all steps proposed by the attending physician to be undertaken are in accord with the desires of the qualified patient.

(b) If the declarant was a qualified patient at least 14 days prior to executing or reexecuting the directive, the directive shall be conclusively presumed, unless revoked, to be the directions of the patient regarding the withholding or withdrawal of life-sustaining procedures. No physician, and no licensed health professional acting under the direction of a physician, shall be criminally or civilly liable for failing to effectuate the directive of the qualified patient pursuant to this subdivision. A failure by a physician to effectuate the directive of a qualified patient pursuant to this division shall constitute unprofessional conduct if the physician refuses to make the necessary arrangements, or fails to take the necessary steps, to effect the transfer of the qualified patient to another physician who will effectuate the directive of the qualified patient.

(c) If the declarant becomes a qualified patient subsequent to executing the directive, and has not subsequently reexecuted the directive, the attending physician may give weight to the directive as evidence of the patient's directions regarding the withholding or withdrawal of life-sustaining procedures and may consider other factors, such as information from the affected family or the nature of the patient's illness, injury, or disease, in determining whether the totality of circumstances known to the attending physician justify effectuating the directive. No physician, and no licensed health professional acting under the direction of a physician, shall be criminally or civilly liable for failing to effectuate the directive of the qualified patient pursuant to this subdivision.

7192. (a) The withholding or withdrawal of life-sustaining procedures from a qualified patient in accordance with the provisions of this chapter shall not, for any purpose, constitute a suicide.

(b) The making of a directive pursuant to Section 7188 shall not restrict, inhibit, or impair in any manner the sale, procurement, or issuance of any policy of life insurance, nor shall it be deemed to modify the terms of an existing policy of life insurance. No policy of life insurance shall be legally impaired or invalidated in any manner by the withholding or withdrawal of life-sustaining procedures from an insured qualified patient, notwithstanding any term of the policy to the contrary.

(c) No physician, health facility, or other health provider, and no health care service plan, insurer issuing disability insurance, self-insured employee welfare benefit plan, or nonprofit hospital service plan, shall require any person to execute a directive as a condition for being insured for, or receiving, health care services.

7193. Nothing in this chapter shall impair or supersede any legal right or legal responsibility which any person may have to effect the withholding or withdrawal of life-sustaining procedures in any lawful manner. In such respect the provisions of this chapter are cumulative.

7194. Any person who willfully conceals, cancels, defaces, obliterates, or damages the directive of another without such declarant's consent shall be guilty of a misdemeanor. Any person who, except where justified or excused by law, falsifies or forges the directive of another, or willfully conceals or withholds personal knowledge of a revocation as provided in Section 7189, with the intent to cause a withholding or withdrawal of life-sustaining procedures contrary to the wishes of the declarant, and thereby, because of any such act, directly causes life-sustaining procedures to be withheld or withdrawn and death to thereby be hastened, shall be subject to prosecution for unlawful homicide as provided in Chapter 1 (commencing with Section 187) of Title 8 of Part 1 of the Penal Code.

7195. Nothing in this chapter shall be construed to condone, authorize, or approve mercy killing, or to permit any affirmative or deliberate act or omission to end life other than to permit the natural process of dying as provided in this chapter.

SEC. 2. If any provision of this act or the application thereof to any person or circumstances is held invalid, such invalidity shall not affect other provisions or applications of the act which can be given effect without the invalid provision or application, and to this end the provisions of this act are severable.

SEC. 3. Notwithstanding Section 2231 of the Revenue and Taxation Code, there shall be no reimbursement pursuant to this section nor shall there be any appropriation made by this act because the Legislature recognizes that during any legislative session a variety of changes to laws relating to crimes and infractions may cause both increased and decreased costs to local government entities and school districts which, in the aggregate, do not result in significant identifiable cost changes.

Appendix G

A Modification of the California Natural Death Act

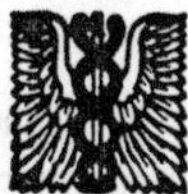

SOCIETY FOR THE RIGHT TO DIE

in support of legislation for death with dignity

250 West 57th Street, New York, N.Y. 10019 • (212) 246-6973

SIDNEY D. ROSOFF, ESQ., PRESIDENT MARCH 1977

RIGHT TO DIE ACT

A MODIFICATION OF THE CALIFORNIA NATURAL DEATH ACT

PROPOSED BY THE SOCIETY FOR THE RIGHT TO DIE

1. PURPOSE AND FINDINGS. The Legislature finds that:

Adult persons have the fundamental right to control the decisions relating to the rendering of their own medical care, including the decision to have life-sustaining procedures withheld or withdrawn in instances of a terminal condition.

Modern medical technology has made possible the prolongation of the dying process beyond natural limits. Such prolongation of the dying process for persons with a terminal condition may cause loss of patient dignity and unnecessary pain and suffering, while providing nothing medically necessary or beneficial to the patient.

There exists considerable uncertainty in the medical and legal professions as to the legality of terminating the use or application of life-sustaining procedures where the patient has voluntarily and in sound mind evidenced a desire that such procedures be withheld or withdrawn.

In recognition of the dignity and privacy which patients have a right to expect, the Legislature hereby declares that the laws of the State of __________ shall recognize the right of an adult person to make a written declaration instructing his or her physician to withhold or withdraw life-sustaining procedures in the event of a terminal condition.

2. DEFINITIONS. The following definitions shall govern the construction of this chapter:

(a) "Attending physician" means the physician selected by, or assigned to, the patient who has primary responsibility for the treatment and care of the patient.

(b) "Declaration" means a witnessed document in writing, voluntarily executed by the declarant in accordance with the requirements of Section 3 of this article.

The declaration, or a copy of the declaration, shall be made part of the patient's medical records.

(c) "Life-sustaining procedure" means any medical procedure or intervention which, when applied to a qualified patient, would serve only to prolong the dying process and where, in the judgment of the attending physician, death will occur whether or not such procedures are utilized. "Life-sustaining procedure" shall not include the administration of medication or the performance of any medical procedure deemed necessary to provide comfort care.

(d) "Physician" means a physician or surgeon licensed by the Board of Medical Examiners of the State of ____________.

(e) "Qualified patient" means a patient diagnosed and certified in writing to be afflicted with a terminal condition by two physicians who have personally examined the patient, one of whom shall be the attending physician.

3. <u>DECLARATION</u>. Any adult person may execute a declaration directing the withholding or withdrawal of life-sustaining procedures in a terminal condition. The declaration shall be signed by the declarant in the presence of two subscribing witnesses. The declaration shall be substantially in the following form:

<u>DECLARATION</u>

Declaration made this ___ day of _____ (month, year). I ________________, being of sound mind, willfully, and voluntarily make known my desire that my dying shall not be artificially prolonged under the circumstances set forth below, do hereby declare:

If at any time I should have an incurable injury, disease, or illness certified to be a terminal condition by two physicians who have personally examined me, one of whom shall be my attending physician, and the physicians have determined that my death will occur whether or not life-sustaining procedures are utilized and where the application of life-sustaining procedures would serve only to artificially prolong the dying process, I direct that such procedures be withheld or withdrawn, and that I be permitted to die naturally with only the administration of medication or the performance of any medical procedure deemed necessary to provide me with comfort care.

In the absence of my ability to give directions regarding the use of such life-sustaining procedures, it is my intention that this declaration shall be honored by my family and physician(s) as the final expression of my legal right to refuse medical or surgical treatment and accept the consequences from such refusal.

I understand the full import of this declaration and I am emotionally and mentally competent to make this declaration.

Signed________________

City, County and State of Residence____________________________

The declarant has been personally known to me and I believe him or her to be of sound mind.

Witness_______________

Witness_______________

4. REVOCATION OF DECLARATION. A declaration may be revoked at any time by the declarant, without regard to his or her mental state or competency, by any of the following methods:

(a) By being canceled, obliterated, or burnt, torn, or otherwise destroyed by the declarant or by some person in his or her presence and by his or her direction.

(b) By a written revocation of the declarant expressing his or her interest to revoke, signed and dated by the declarant. The attending physician shall record in the patient's medical record the time and date when he or she received notification of the written revocation.

(c) By a verbal expression by the declarant of his or her intent to revoke the declaration. Such revocation shall become effective upon communication to the attending physician by the declarant or by a person acting on behalf of the declarant. The attending physician shall record in the patient's medical record the time, date and place of the revocation and the time, date and place, if different, of when he or she received notification of the revocation.

5. No physician or health facility which, when acting in accordance with the requirements of this chapter, causes the withholding or withdrawal of life-sustaining procedures from a qualified patient, shall be subject to civil liability therefrom. No licensed health professional, acting under the direction of a physician, who participates in the withholding or withdrawal of life-sustaining procedures in accordance with the provisions of this chapter shall be subject to any civil liability. No physician, or licensed health care professional acting under the direction of a physician, who participates in the withholding of withdrawal of life-sustaining procedures in accordance with the provisions of this chapter shall be guilty of any criminal act or of unprofessional conduct.

6. Prior to effecting a withholding or withdrawal of life-sustaining procedures from a qualified patient pursuant to the declaration, the attending physician shall detemine that the declaration complies with Section 3, and, if the patient is mentally competent, that the declaration and all steps proposed by the attending physician are in accord with the desires of the qualified patient. No physician, and no licensed health care professional acting under the direction of a physician, shall be criminally or civilly liable for failing to effectuate the declaration of a qualified patient pursuant to this subdivision. A failure by a physician to effectuate the declaration of a qualified patient pursuant to this subdivision shall constitute unprofessional conduct if the physican refuses to make the necessary arrangements, or fails to take the necessary steps, to effect the transfer of the qualified patient to another physician who will effectuate the declaration of the qualified patient.

7. INSURANCE. The making of a declaration pursuant to Section 3 shall not restrict, inhibit or impair in any manner the sale, procurement, or issuance of any policy of life insurance, nor shall it be deemed to modify the terms of an existing policy of life insurance. No policy of life insurance shall be legally impaired or invalidated in any manner by the withholding or withdrawal of life-sustaining procedures from an insured qualified patient, notwithstanding any term of the policy to the contrary.

No physician, health facility, or other health provider, and no health care service plan, insurer issuing disability insurance, self-insured employee welfare benefit plan, or nonprofit hospital plan, shall require any person to execute a declaration as a condition for being insured for, or receiving, health care services.

8. Nothing in this chapter shall impair or supercede any legal right or legal responsibility which any person may have to effect the withholding or withdrawal of life-sustaining procedures in any lawful manner. In such respect the provisions of this chapter are cumulative.

9. CRIMINAL LIABILITY. Any person who willfully conceals, cancels, defaces, obliterates, or damages the declaration of another without such declarant's consent shall be guilty of a misdemeanor. Any person who falsifies or forges the declaration of another, or willfully conceals or withholds personal knowledge of a revocation as provided in Section 4, with the intent to cause a withholding or withdrawal of life-sustaining procedures contrary to the wishes of the declarant, and thereby, because of any such act, directly causes life-sustaining procedures to be withheld or withdrawn and death to thereby be hastened, shall be subject to prosecution for unlawful homicide.

10. SEVERABILITY. If any provision of this act or the application thereof to any person or circumstances is held invalid, such invalidity shall not affect other provisions of applications of the act which can be given effect without the invalid provision or application, and to this end the provisions of this act are severable.

Appendix H

Letter of Transmittal: Legislation Survey

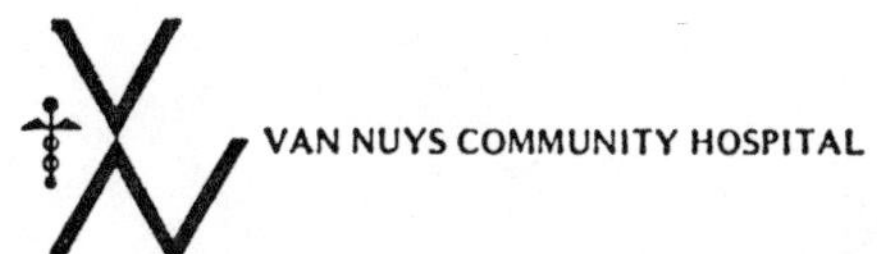

14433 Emelita Street · Van Nuys, California 91401 · Phone [213] 787-1511

October 11, 1977

Gentlemen:

I am currently preparing a doctoral dissertation entitled: "A Study of the Hospice Movement in the United States and Canada." Part of the research involves determining what legislation pertaining to hospices, terminally ill, euthanasia, and related topics exists and is pending at the State level in the United States and at the Provincial level in Canada.

I am requesting the above information as it pertains to your State (Province). Could you forward this request to the appropriate person/agency who would be most knowledgeable in this rather specialized area of interest?

If you are interested in the results of this research, I would be most happy to supply you with a summary at completion. Merely indicate this request by return mail.

Thank you for your cooperation in furthering the interests of scientific investigation.

Cordially,

Kenneth P. Cohen
Administrator
KPC/br

P.S. Definition of Hospice: A program which provides palliative and supportive care for terminally ill patients and their families, either directly or on a consulting basis with the patient's physician or another community agency such as a visiting nurse association. Originally a medieval name for a way station for pilgrims and travelers where they could be replenished, refreshed, and cared for; used here for an organized program of care for people going through life's last station. The whole family is considered the unit of care and care extends through the mourning process. Emphasis is placed on symptom control and preparation for and support before and after death, full scope health services being provided by an organized interdisciplinary team available on a twenty-four hours-a-day, seven-days-a-week basis.*

* U.S. Congress, House, Committee on Interstate and Foreign Commerce, Sub-Committee on Health and the Environment, A Discursive Dictionary of Health Care, February 1976, 94th Congress, 2nd Session.

Appendix I

Letter of Transmittal: Hospice Survey

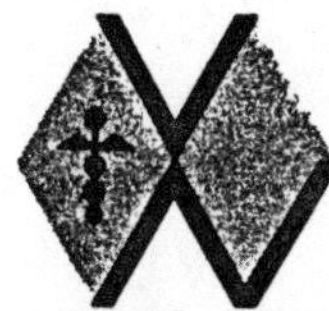

VAN NUYS COMMUNITY HOSPITAL

14433 Emelita Street • Van Nuys, California 91401 Phone [213] 787-1511

January 10, 1978

Dear Administrator:

Your organization has been identified as being a hospice or as a hospice in process of development. I am currently preparing a doctoral dissertation entitled "A Study of the Hospice Movement in the United States and Canada." In order that the research may be complete I need to identify hospice programs and present certain information about each of the programs. A publisher has indicated interest in adapting the dissertation to a book to be published hopefully in late 1978.

If your hospice wishes to be mentioned in the dissertation and the book, I will need certain information from you which is contained in the enclosed questionnaire. The questionnaire has been designed so that you need spend only a few minutes of your valuable time in preparation. Please return in the enclosed stamped envelope by February 3, 1978.

As soon as the publication date is established I shall notify you of the details of publication. This is a mechanism for your hospice to gain recognition nationally with very little investment of time on your part.

Thank you for your cooperation in furthering the interests of scientific investigation.

Cordially,

Kenneth P. Cohen

Kenneth P. Cohen
Administrator

KPC:cen

Appendix J

Questionnaire: Hospice Survey

HOSPICE SURVEY

1. Organization Name____________________________________
2. Mailing Address__________________City__________State_____Zip_____
3. Office Address__________________City__________State_____Zip_____
4. Phone No. (   )__________________
   area   phone
5. Director/Administrator____________________Title____________
6. Person responding to Questionnaire____________________Title____________
7. May I use this information in the dissertation/book? (write Yes or No)__________
8. Ownership of Hospice (check all that apply). Corporation ( ) Partnership ( )
   Proprietorship ( ) Not Incorporated Group ( ) Non-Profit ( )
   Investor Owned ( ) Public Owned: City, County, Etc. ( )
   Other ( ) specify____________________
9. Please check all programs you provide or plan to provide:
   a) Inpatient Palliative Care ( ) No. beds______
   b) Home Palliative Care ( )
   c) Consulting & Referral Services ( )
   d) Bereavement Follow up Services ( )
   e) Teaching or instruction (i.e., medical students, secondary school, nurses, public, volunteers) ( ).
   f) Other (specify)________ ________________( )
10. Services offered or to be offered:
    Medical ( ) Homemaker ( ) Social Services ( )
    Nursing ( ) Lay Volunteer ( ) Other (specify)____________
    Counseling ( ) Spiritual ( ) ________________( )
11. Date your program began or is expected to begin____________________
12. In number days per week and hours per day, indicate normal visiting times____/____
    days hours
13. What age restrictions for visitors?____________________________
14. What is your unit of Care? (check one) Patient ( ) Family ( )
    Patient and Family ( ) Other ( ) specify____________________
15. What % of your patients come from within the following distances from your facility?
    Less than 10 miles _____%
    10 but less than 30 miles _____%
    30 but less than 50 miles _____%
    50 but less than 100 miles _____%
    100 or more miles _____%
16. Population served:
    Less than 100,000 ( )
    100,000 - 500,000 ( )
    500,000 - 1,000,000 ( )
    1,000,000 and over ( )
17. Do you provide home care services 24 hours per day, seven days per week?
    Yes ( ) No ( ) If no, what basis?____________________
    How many patients can you serve?________ If you don't provide home care services, are you planning to provide in future? Yes ( ) No ( )
18. For inpatients, what is average length of stay? _____days. Avg. Daily Census_______
19. How many volunteers are involved in your program?____________________
20. What is the average number hours of service each volunteer provides?__________
21. What training do volunteers undergo?__________________________
22. How many full time equivalent employees (35 hrs. or more per week):

Personnel Category	Full-Time Equivalents	Personnel Category	Full-Time Equivalents
Registered Nurse	______	Clergy	______
Licensed Practical/Vocational Nurse	______	Administrative	______
Social Worker	______	Housekeeping	______
Physician	______	Other (specify)______	______

HOSPICE SURVEY

23. Approximately what % of your patients are admitted with a diagnosis of:
    - Cancer ____%
    - Kidney ____%
    - Heart Disease ____%
    - Other (specify)____________ ____%

    100 %

24. What % of your patients are:
    - Under 18 years of age ____%
    - Between 18 and 64 ____%
    - 65 and over ____%

25. For third party reimbursement, how are your beds classified?
    - Acute hospital ____
    - Skilled nursing ____
    - Intermediate nursing ____
    - Chronic Disease ____
    - Other (specify)____________

26. What is % breakdown of total revenue by payor?
    - Medicare ____%
    - Medicaid ____%
    - Commercial Insurance ____%
    - Self Pay ____%
    - Philanthropy ____%
    - Other (specify)____________ ____%

    100 %

27. Sources of funding:
    - Foundations ( )
    - Federal Grant(s) ( )
    - State Government ( )
    - County ( )
    - Church ( )
    - Other (specify)____________ ( )

28. Do you provide special overnight accommodations for families of patients?
    Yes ( ) No ( ) If yes, please describe ____________________

29. Additional Comments?____________________

Thank you for your time. You have been of tremendous assistance. Please return this questionnaire by February 3, 1978 in the enclosed envelope to:

Kenneth P. Cohen, Administrator
Van Nuys Community Hospital
14433 Emelita Street
Van Nuys, California 91401

Bibliography

Ajemian, Ina. "An Oral Morphine Mixture for Intractable Pain." *Canadian Family Physician* 23 (1977): 1,506–7.

Allen, George R. *The Graduate Student's Guide to Theses and Dissertations: A Practical Manual for Writing and Research*. San Francisco: Jossey-Bass, 1973.

Alsofrom, J. "Hospice Way of Dying—At Home with Friends and Family." *American Medical News* 20 (February 21, 1977): 7–9.

American Bar Association. *Report of the Committee on Medicine and Law* 11, forum 300 (1976): 311.

American Cancer Society. *Proceedings of the American Cancer Society's National Conference on Human Values and Cancer, Atlanta, Georgia, June 22–24, 1972*. New York: American Cancer Society, 1973.

American Health Congress. *Death and Dying*. Chicago: American Health Congress, 1973. Cassette tape recordings available through the American Hospital Association, Chicago.

American Medical Association. *AMA Council Guideline for Physicians on Euthanasia*. Chicago: American Medical Association, 1973.

American Medical Association. "The Physician and the Dying Patient." Report of the Judicial Council, American Medical Association, adopted by the AMA House of Delegates, December 1973. Mimeographed.

Annas, George J. "The Legal Aspects of a Patient Care Classification System." *The Hospital Medical Staff* 5 (February 1976): 12–18.

__________. *The Rights of Hospital Patients: The Basic ACLU Guide to a Hospital Patient's Rights*. New York: Avon Books, 1975.

Ariés, Philippe. "A Moment That Has Lost Its Meaning." *Prism* 3 (June 1975): 27 ff.

Ashley, Beth. "A Dying Man Tells How Hospice Helps." *Independent-Journal*, November 15, 1976.

Bachmann, Charles C. *Ministering to the Grief Sufferer*. Englewood Cliffs, New Jersey: Prentice-Hall, 1964.

Bacon, Francis. "Of Death." *Essaies of Sir Francis Bacon*. London: John Beale, 1612.

Bailey, David. "Requiem in Venice." *Prism* 3 (June 1975): 30–3.

Baillie, J. *And the Life Everlasting*. New York: Scribner, 1933.

Bard, Morton. "The Psychological Impact of Cancer and Cancer Surgery." *Proceedings of the American Cancer Society's National Conference on Human Values and Cancer*. Atlanta: American Cancer Society, 1972.

Bates, Richard C. "It's *Our* Right to Pull the Plug." *Medical Economics,* May 16, 1977, pp. 162–166.

Becker, Howard and Bruner, D. K. "Attitudes Toward Death and the Dead and Some Possible Causes of Ghost Fear." *Mental Hygiene* 15 (1931): 828–37.

Behnke, John A. and Bok, Sissela, eds. *Dilemmas of Euthanasia.* New York: Anchor Press, 1975.

Bell, Rev. Howard. "Eight Weeks to Live, Eight Weeks to Die." *Y Circulator.* Edited by Charlotte Himber. New York: National Board of YMCAs, n.d., pp. 3–4.

Bergen, Richard P. "Management of Terminal Illness." *JAMA* 229 (September 2, 1974): 1,352–3.

Bernstein, Barton E. "Lawyer and Counselor as an Interdisciplinary Team: Interfacing for the Terminally Ill." *Death Education* 1 (Fall 1977): 277–91.

Black, P. McL. "Focusing on Some of the Ethical Problems Associated with Death and Dying." *Geriatrics* 31 (January 1976): 138–41.

Black's Law Dictionary. 4th ed. St. Paul: West Publishing Co., 1968.

Blue Cross and Blue Shield Associations. "Initial Statement on Hospice Care and Payment for Hospice Services." Approved November 8, 1978 by the boards of the Blue Cross and Blue Shield Associations.

Brim, Orville G., Jr. et al., eds. *The Dying Patient.* New York: Russell Sage Foundation, 1970.

Brown, Norman K.; Brown, Maria A.; and Thompson, Donovan. "Decision Making for the Terminally Ill Patient." *Cancer: The Behavioral Dimensions.* Edited by J. W. Cullen, B. H. Fox, and R. N. Isom. Bethesda, Maryland: HEW, Public Health Service, National Institutes of Health, National Cancer Institute, HEW Publication No. (NIH) 76-1074, n.d., pp. 3–91 to 3–104.

Budge, E. A. Wallis. *The Book of the Dead.* New Hyde Park, N.Y.: University Books, 1960.

Bullough, Vern L. "The Banal and Costly Funeral." *The Humanist* 4 (1960): 213–18.

Burch, G. E. "Of the Family of the Sick." *American Heart Journal* 92 (September 1976): 405.

Burkhalter, P. K. "Fostering Staff Sensitivity to the Dying Patient." *Supervisor Nurse* 6 (April 1975): 55–59.

Caldwell, J. R. "One Hundred Deaths in Practice." *Journal of the Royal College of General Practitioners* 21 (1971): 460.

California Medical Association. *A Proposal for Care of the Terminally Ill: Report to the Council* by the Committee on Evolving Trends in Society Affecting Life, Resolution No. 85-77, August 5, 1977, Laurens P. White, Chairman.

Canada, Health and Welfare, Health Programs Branch. Personal letter from Robert H. Lennox, Senior Consultant, Child & Adult Health, Health Consultants, November 1, 1977.

"Cancer Patients' Organization Helps Them Deal with Problems of Living." *JAMA* 235 (May 10, 1976): 2,065–67.

Cancer Statistics, 1977. New York: American Cancer Society, 1977.

Canvin, R. W. and Newell, J. M. "Care of the Dying in Exeter." *Nursing Times* 71 (June 12, 1975): 942–3.

Capron, A. M. and Kass, L. R. "A Statutory Definition of the Standards for Determining Human Death: An Appraisal and a Proposal." *University of Pennsylvania Law Review* 121 (1972): 87–118.

"Care of the Dying Patient." *Journal of Family Practice* 3 (October 1976): 547–55.

Carlozzi, Carl G. *Death and Contemporary Man: The Crisis of Terminal Illness*. Grand Rapids, Michigan: William B. Eerdmans, 1968.

Carroll, Patrick A. "Who Speaks for Incompetent Patients? The Case of Joseph Saikewicz." *Trustee* 31 (December 1978): 19–24.

Castiglioni, Arturo. *A History of Medicine*. 2nd ed. Translated and edited by E. B. Krumbhaar. New York: Knopf, 1958.

"Cause of Death: Bureaucracy." *Prism* 3 (June 1975): 22–6 ff.

Changing Attitudes Toward Euthanasia: Excerpts From Papers Presented at the 8th Annual Euthanasia Conference. New York: The Euthanasia Educational Council, 1975.

Chapelle, Dickey. "Water War in Viet Nam." *National Geographic* 129 (February 1966): 272–96.

Charles, Eleanor. "A Hospice For the Terminally Ill." *New York Times*, March 13, 1977.

Cheatum, Lynne. "Hospice Here Helps the Dying." *Kansas City Star*, October 5, 1977.

———. "Joint Project Aids Terminally Ill Patients." Reprint. *Kansas City Star*, n.d. (approximately September 25, 1977).

Christensen, Robert A. "When Each Extra Day Counts." *American Journal of Nursing* 77 (May 1977): 853.

Clothier, Florence. "Euthanasia—the Physician's Dilemma." Mimeographed. New York: The Euthanasia Educational Council, 1972.

"'Code' or 'No Code'." *The Bulletin*, Los Angeles County Medical Association, February 16, 1978, p. 16.

Coffin, Margaret M. *Death in Early America*. New York: Thomas Nelson, 1976.

Cohen, Kenneth P. "A Study of the Hospice Movement in the United States and Canada." Ph.D. dissertation, California Western University, 1978.

Cook, S. S. *Children and Dying: An Exploration and a Selective Professional Bibliography*. New York: Health Sciences, 1973.

Cotter, Z. M. "Institutional Care of the Terminally Ill." *Hospital Progress* 52 (June 1971): 42–8.

Craven, Joan and Wald, Florence S. "Hospice Care for Dying Patients." *American Journal of Nursing* 75 (October 1975): 1,816–22.

Criminal Code of Canada. Sections 198, 199, 202, 205, 209, 212.

Crosby, Edwin L. "Hospital." *World Book Encyclopedia*, 1967.

Davidson, Glen W. *Living with Dying*. Minneapolis: Augsberg Publishing House, 1975.

Davis, Richard H., ed. *Dealing with Death*. Los Angeles: Ethel Percy Andrus Gerontology Center, University of Southern California, 1973.

Dawson, Bernard. *The History of Medicine*. London: Lewis, 1931.

Day, Stacey B. *Tuluak and Amaulik: Dialogues on Death and Mourning with the Invit Eskimo of Point Barrow and Wainwright, Alaska*. Minneapolis: University of Minnesota Printing Dept., 1973.

Death and Decisions: Excerpts from Papers at the 7th Annual Euthanasia Conference. New York: Euthanasia Educational Council, 1974.

"Definition of Death." *JAMA* 227 (February 18, 1974): 728.

"A Definition of Irreversible Coma: Report of the Ad Hoc Committee of the Harvard Medical School to Examine the Definition of Brain Death." *JAMA* 205 (August 5, 1968): 337–40.

DeMere, M. et al. "Report on Definition of Death, from Law and Medicine Committee." Chicago: American Bar Association, 1975.

Dobihal, Edward F. "Talk or Terminal Care?" *Connecticut Medicine* 38 (July 1974): 364–67.

"Doctor Charged in Man's Death." *Los Angeles Times,* March 31, 1978, part II, p. 5.

Downie, P. A. "Havens of Peace." *Nursing Times* 69 (August 16, 1973): 1,068–70.

Downing, A. B. ed. *Euthanasia and the Right To Die.* London: Peter Owen, 1969.

Du Bois, Paul. "Hospices: A New Way To Die." Ph.D. dissertation, Cornell University, 1977.

Duff, R. S. and Campbell, A. G. M. "On Deciding the Care of Severely Handicapped or Dying Persons: with Particular Reference to Infants." *Pediatrics* 57 (April 1976, part 1): 487–93.

Eissler, Kurt R. *The Psychiatrist and the Dying Patient.* New York: International Universities Press, 1955.

Elder, R. "Dying in the USA." *International Journal of Nursing Studies* 10 (August 1973): 171–84.

"Elderly Woman Who Fought To Save Her Gangrenous Feet Dies." *Los Angeles Times,* May 2, 1978.

Erickson, Franklin. "Saint Bernard, Great and Saint Bernard, Little." *World Book Encyclopedia,* 1967.

Ersland, Celia. "These Nurses Take Sorrow from Dying." *The Press Democrat* (Santa Rosa, California), November 6, 1977.

The Euthanasia Educational Council. *Death & Decisions: Excerpts from Papers & Discussion at the 7th Annual Euthanasia Conference.* New York: The Euthanasia Educational Council, 1974.

The Euthanasia Educational Council. *Dilemmas of Euthanasia: Excerpts from Papers & Discussion at the 4th Euthanasia Conference.* New York: The Euthanasia Educational Council, 1971.

"Facts About Hospice." Mimeographed. New Haven, Connecticut: Hospice, Inc., October 1977.

Farberow, Norman L. ed. *Taboo Topics.* New York: Atherton Press, 1963.

Farm Bureau Life Insurance Company, West Des Moines, Iowa. Personal letter from Harry J. Solliday, Product Research and Development Analyst, October 2, 1977.

Fatteh, A. "A Lawsuit That Led to a Redefinition of Death." *Journal of Legal Medicine* 1 (July-August 1973): 30–4.

Federal Drug Enforcement Administration. *Drugs of Abuse.* Washington, D.C.: Government Printing Office n.d.

Feifel, Herman. "Death and Dying in Modern America." *Death Education* 1 (Spring 1977): 5–14.

———, ed. *The Meaning of Death.* New York: McGraw-Hill, 1959.

———. *New Meanings of Death.* New York: McGraw-Hill, 1977.

Ferber, Max. "I Cried, But Not for Irma." *Reader's Digest,* April 1976, pp. 92–4.

Fletcher, Joseph. *Morals and Medicine.* Boston: Beacon, 1960.

Fochtman, Marie D. "A Comparative Study of Pediatric Nurses' Attitudes Towards Death." Master's thesis, University of California, Los Angeles, 1971.

"For the Terminally Ill, A Hospital That Cares: St. Christopher's Hospice, London." *Medical World News* 15 (July 19, 1974): 46–7.

Freihofer, P. and Felton, G. "Nursing Behaviours in Bereavement: An Exploratory Study." *Nursing Research* 25 (September-October 1976): 332–7.

Friedman, Emily. "California Hospitals Design Natural Death Act Procedures." *Hospitals* 51 (November 16, 1977): 62–65.

________. "'Natural Death' Laws Cause Hospitals Few Problems." *Hospitals* 52 (May 16, 1978): 124 ff.

Froslid, E. Kenneth. "A Definition of Death," *World Book Year Book*, 1969, p. 407.

Fulton, R. *Death, Grief and Bereavement: A Chronological Bibliography, 1843–1970*. Minneapolis: University of Minnesota, Center For Death Education and Research, 1970.

Fulton, Robert. *Death and Identity*. rev. ed. Bowie, Maryland: Charles Press, 1976.

Garfield, Charles A. and Clark, Rachel O. "Shanti Project: Volunteer Counseling Service for Patients and Families Facing Life-Threatening Illness" *Hospital Forum* 20 (September-October 1977): 4–6.

Garner, Jim. "Palliative Care: It's the Quality of Life Remaining That Matters." *Canadian Medical Association JRNL* 115 (July 17, 1976): 179–80.

Garrett, W. E. "South to Mexico City." *National Geographic* 134 (August 1968): 145–93.

Glaser, Barney and Strauss, Anselm. *Awareness of Dying*. Chicago: Aldine Publishing, 1965.

________. "The Social Loss of Dying Patients." *American Journal of Nursing* 63 (January 1964): 119–21.

Goodman, James. "New Jersey, Death and the Law." *1976 Yearbook, Covering the Year 1975*. New York: Collier, 1975, p. 374.

Gorer, Geoffrey. *Death, Grief, and Mourning in Contemporary Britain*. London: Cresset Press, 1965.

Gould, Donald W. and Snider, Arthur J. "Health and Disease, General Overview." *1976 Britannica Book of the Year, Events of 1975*. Chicago: Encyclopaedia Britannica, 1976.

Gould, Jonathan and Craigmyle, T.D.M.S., eds. *Your Death Warrant? The Implications of Euthanasia—A Medical, Legal and Ethical Study*. Worcester, England: Fowler Wright, 1971.

Group Hospitalization, Inc. (Blue Cross), Washington, D.C. Unpublished study on hospice, n.d.

Hackley, John A. "Full Service Hospice Offers Home, Day, and Inpatient Care." *Hospitals* 51 (November 1, 1977): 84–7.

Halporn, Roberta, comp. and ed. *The Hospice Concept*. Brooklyn: Highly Specialized Promotions, 1977.

Hambly, Wilfred D. "Funeral Customs." *World Book Encyclopedia*, 1967.

Harrington, Michael. *The Other America: Poverty in the U.S.* Baltimore: Penguin Books, 1963.

Hartland, E. Sidney. "Death and Disposal of the Dead." *Encyclopedia of Religion & Ethics*, 1928.

Hatton, Corinne L.; Valente, Sharon M.; and Rink, Alice; eds. *Suicide: Assessment and Intervention*. New York: Appleton-Century-Crofts, 1977.

Headlee, Judith Anne. "Let Grieving Go." *The Single Parent* 18 (October 1975): 12–16.

Hearing Transcript on "No Code" orders held September 21, 1977 by the Chief Medical Examiner-Coroner Committee of the Board of Supervisors, Los Angeles County Board of Supervisors, the Honorable Baxter Ward, presiding.

Heifetz, Milton D. with Mangel, Charles. *The Right To Die: A Neurosurgeon Speaks of Death with Candor*. New York: Putnam's Sons, 1975.

Hertz, Robert. *Death and the Right Hand.* Aberdeen, England: University Press, 1960.

Hillhaven Hospice Medical Newsletter, Hillhaven Hospice, Tucson, Arizona, vol. I, no. 1.

Hines, William. "London Hospice Dedicated to Serving the Terminally Ill." *Los Angeles Times,* December 9, 1977.

Hinton, John. *Dying*. Middlesex, England: Penguin Books, Ltd., 1967.

Hocart, A. M. "Death Customs." *Encyclopedia of the Social Sciences*. Edited by Seligman and Johnson. New York: MacMillan, 1931.

Holden, C. "Hospices: For the Dying, Relief from Pain and Fear." *Science* 193 (July 30, 1976): 389–91.

"Hospice." An Interview with William M. Lamers, Jr., Medical Director, Hospice of Marin. *Thanatos,* March 1977, pp. 6–11.

"Hospice Care Covered." *Modern Healthcare* 8 (April 1978): 30.

"Hospice Care—A New Concept For the Care of the Terminally Ill and Their Families." Workshop at UCLA Extension, Los Angeles, April 8–9, 1978.

"Hospice Concept Continues to Grow in California." *CHA Insight* 3 (December 28, 1977), 2 pp.

"The Hospice Movement." Management Services Special Report. Unpublished. Newport Beach, California: Advanced Health Systems, Inc., 1977.

"Hospice Provides Home Care For Terminally Ill." *American Journal of Nursing* 74 (April 1974): 717.

Hospital Statistics, 1977 Edition. Chicago: American Hospital Association, 1977.

"The 'How To' of Hospice Care." Third National Hospice Symposium, Dominican College Campus, San Rafael, California, May 26–28, 1977.

Hudson, Robert P. "How Real Is Our Reverence for Life?" *Prism* 3 (June 1975): 19–21 ff.

Hume, Edgar E. *Medical Work of Knights Hospitallers of Saint John of Jerusalem*. Baltimore: Johns Hopkins Press, 1940.

Indiana State Board of Health. "The Hospice: Care for People with Terminal Illness." Indianapolis: Indiana State Board of Health, 1977.

Ingles, T. "St. Christopher's Hospice." *Nursing Outlook* 22 (December 1974): 759–63.

Inquest Transcript Held on the Body of One Raymond S. Oden, Los Angeles, Calif., August 30–31, 1977.

Jackson, Edgar. *Understanding Grief.* Nashville: Abingdon, 1957.

Jakobovits, Immanuel. *Jewish Medical Ethics*. New York: Bloch, 1959.

Judd, Leda R. "Hospices—A Background Paper." Unpublished report prepared for HEW, n.d.

Kalish, R. A. "Death and Bereavement: A Bibliography." *Human Relations* 13 (1965): 118–41.

Kalish, Richard A. "The Aged and the Dying Process: The Inevitable Decisions." *Journal of Social Issues* 21 (1965): 87–96.

__________. "Social Distance and the Dying." *Community Mental Health Journal* 2 (1966): 152–5.

Kantor, Alice. "Focus on Hospice: Improving the Quality of Life That Remains." *St. Luke's Hospital Center News* (New York), n.d., pp. 3–4.

Kaplan, R. P. "Euthanasia Legislation: A Survey and a Model Act." *American Journal of Law Medicine* 2 (Summer 1976): 41–99.

"Karen Ann Quinlan Passes Third Year in Coma." *Health Care Week,* April 24, 1978, p. 6.

Kast, Shelia. "Hospice: A Way To Combat the Loneliness in a Loved One's Final Days of Life." *The Washington Star,* November 28, 1977.

Kastenbaum, Robert and Costa, Paul T., Jr. "Psychological Perspectives on Death." *Annual Review of Psychology* 28 (1977): 225–49.

Katz, Jay and Capron, Alexander M. *Catastrophic Diseases: Who Decides What?* New York: Russell Sage Foundation, 1975.

Kelly, Francis B. *1977–1978 Nationwide Hospital Insurance Billing Directory.* Los Angeles: Francis B. Kelly & Associates, 1977.

Kerstein, Morris D. "Caring For the Terminally Ill: A Hospice." *American Journal of Psychiatry* 129 (August 1972): 237–8.

Klutch, Murray, "Hospices for Terminally Ill Patients: The California Experience." *Western Journal of Medicine* 129 (July 1978): 82–4.

Kohl, Marvin, ed. *Beneficent Euthanasia.* Buffalo, New York: Prometheus Books, 1975.

Kohn, J. "Hospice Building Speaks on Many Emotional Levels to Patient, Family." *Modern Healthcare* 5 (October 1976): 56–7.

Kohn, Judith. "Hospice Movement Provides Humane Alternative for Terminally Ill Patients." *Modern Healthcare* 6 (September 1976): 26–8.

Kolbe, Richard. "Inside the English Hospice." *Hospitals* 51 (July 1, 1977): 65–7.

Koop, C. Everett. *The Right To Live: The Right To Die.* Wheaton, Illinois: Tyndale House, 1976.

Koster, Mary. "Should 'Brain Death' Definition Be Law? No." *Health Care Week* 1 (February 13, 1978): 9.

Krant, M. D. et al. "The Role of a Hospital-Based Psychosocial Unit in Terminal Cancer Illness and Bereavement." *Journal of Chronic Diseases* 29 (February 1976): 115–27.

Krant, Melvin J. *Dying and Dignity: The Meaning and Control of a Personal Death.* Springfield, Illinois: Charles C. Thomas, 1974.

Kron, Joan. "Designing a Better Place To Die." *New York,* March 1, 1976, pp. 43–9.

Kubler-Ross, Elisabeth. *Death: The Final Stage of Growth.* Englewood Cliffs, New Jersey: Prentice-Hall, 1975.

———. *On Death and Dying.* New York: Macmillan, 1969.

———. *Living with Dying.* Speech sponsored by Power Within, Lobero Theater, Santa Barbara, California, October 4, 1977.

Kutscher, A. H. and Kutscher, A. H., Jr. *A Bibliography of Books on Death, Bereavement, Loss and Grief.* New York: Health Sciences, 1970.

Kutscher, Austin H., ed. *Death and Bereavement.* Springfield, Illinois: Charles C Thomas, 1969.

Lack, Sylvia. "I Want To Die While I'm Still Alive." *Death Education* 1 (Summer 1977): 165–76.

Lack, Sylvia. "Philosophy and Organization of a Hospice Program." Unpublished paper, n.d.

———. Mimeographed. Private instruction sheet prepared by Medical Director, Hospice Inc., New Haven, Connecticut, n.d.

Lack, Sylvia and Buckingham, Robert W., III. *First American Hospice: Three Years of Home Care*. New Haven: Hospice, Inc., 1978.

Lamerton, Richard. *Care of the Dying*. Westport, Connecticut: Technomic Publishing Co., Inc., 1976.

__________. "The Need For Hospices." *Nursing Times* 71 (January 23, 1975): 155–7.

Lee, James Marvin. "The Nurse and the Terminally Ill Patient: An Experimental Study." Ph.D. dissertation, Texas Tech University, 1972.

Legislative Manual: Death with Dignity. New York: The Society for the Right To Die, 1976.

Legislative Manual, 1978. New York: Society for the Right to Die, 1978.

Legislative Newsletter. New York: Society for the Right to Die, Summer 1977.

Lescoe, R. J. "Legislative Proposals for Death and Dignity." *Journal of Legal Medicine* 3 (September 1975): 34–5.

Lestz, Paula. "A Committee To Decide the Quality of Life." *American Journal of Nursing* 77 (May 1977): 862–4.

Levin, David L. et al. *Cancer Rates and Risks*. 2nd ed. HEW Publication No. (NIH) 75-691. Washington, D.C.: U.S. Government Printing Office, 1974.

Lewis, Tony. "Dorothy Krahl: Hospice Gave Them an Alternate to an Impersonal Death." *Twin Cities Times*, April 27, 1977.

Lewis, Tony. "Hospice of Marin: Caring For the Terminally Ill at Home." *Twin Cities Times*, March 30, 1977.

Libman, Joan. "Hospice Movement Stresses Care for the Terminally Ill." *Wall Street Journal*, March 28, 1978.

Liegner, Leonard M. "St. Christopher's Hospice, 1974: Care of the Dying Patient," *JAMA* 234 (December 8, 1975): 1,047–8.

Life and Death and Medicine: A Scientific American Book. San Francisco: W. H. Freeman & Co., 1973.

"Life and Death in the Palliative Care Unit: Montreal's Royal Victoria Hospital." *Dimensions in Health Service* 52 (September 1975): 22.

Lindemann, E. "Symptomatology and Management of Acute Grief." *American Journal of Psychiatry* 101 (1944): 141.

Lipman, A. C. "Drug Therapy in Terminally Ill Patients." *American Journal of Hospital Pharmacy* 32 (March 1975): 270–6.

Longo, D. R. and Darr, K. "Hospital Care For the Terminally Ill: A Model Program." *Hospital Progress* 59 (March 1978): 62–5, 84.

Lucente, F. E. "Thanatology: A Study of 100 Deaths." *Transactions of the American Academy of Ophthalmology and Otolaryngology* 76 (March-April 1972): 334–9.

MacEachern, Malcolm T. *Hospital Organization and Management*. rev. 3rd. ed. Berwyn, Illinois: Physicians Record Co., 1962.

MacLeish, Kenneth. "Singapore, Reluctant Nation." *National Geographic* 130 (August 1966): 268–300.

Maguire, Daniel C. *Death by Choice*. Garden City, New York: Doubleday, 1974.

Marshall, J. G. "Annotated Bibliography: A Selected List of Children's Books Relating to Death." *Omega* 2 (1971): 41–5.

Martinson, Ida M. "Why Don't We Let Them Die at Home?" *RN*, January 1976.

Mayer, Milton. "On Death." *The Great Ideas Today, 1965*. Edited by Robert M. Hutchins and Mortimer J. Adler. Chicago: Encyclopaedia Britannica, Inc., 1965.

McCarthy, D. G. "Should Catholic Hospitals Sponsor Hospices?" *Hospital Progress* 57 (December 1976): 61–5.

McGeveran, William A. "A Right To Die?" *1977 Yearbook*. New York: Collier, 1976.

McGibony, John R. *Principles of Hospital Administration*. 2nd ed. New York: Putnam's, 1969.

McKeighen, Rosemary J. "A Study of Expectancy and Family Grief Reactions." Master's thesis, University of California-Los Angeles, 1967.

McNulty, B. J. "Domicilliary Care of the Dying: Some Problems Encountered." *Nursing Mirror* 136 (May 18, 1973): 29–30.

________. "St. Christopher's Outpatients." *American Journal of Nursing* 71 (December 1971): 2,328–30.

Meek, H. B. "Hotel." *World Book Encyclopedia*, 1967.

Melzack, R.; Ofiesh, J. G.; and Mount, B. M. "The Brompton Mixture: Effects on Pain in Cancer Patients." *Canadian Medical Association Journal* 115 (July 17, 1976): 125–8.

Mervyn, Frances. "The Plight of Dying Patients in Hospitals ." *American Journal of Nursing* 71 (October 1971): 1,988–90.

Mihanovich, C. S. "Euthanasia." *World Book Encyclopedia*, 1967.

Mitford, Jessica. *The American Way of Death*. New York: Simon & Schuster, 1963.

Mitra, D. N. "Mourning Customs and Modern Life in Bengal." *American Journal of Sociology* 52 (1947): 309–11.

Mount, Balfour et al. "Death and Dying: Attitudes in a Teaching Hospital." *Urology* 4 (December 1974): 741–7.

Mount, Balfour. "Death—A Part of Life?" *Crux* 11 (1973–1974): 3–6.

________. "Improving the Canadian Way of Dying." *The Ontario Psychologist* 7 (June 1975): 19.

________. "The Problem of Caring for the Dying in a General Hospital: The Palliative Care Unit As a Possible Solution." *Canadian Medical Association Journal* 115 (July 17, 1976): 119–21.

Mount, B. M. et al. "Use of the Brompton Mixture in Treating the Chronic Pain of Malignant Disease." *Canadian Medical Association Journal* 115 (July 17, 1976): 122–4.

Munk, William. *Euthanasia: Or Medical Treatment in Aid of an Easy Death*. London: Longman, Green & Co., 1887.

Nash, Mary Louise; Connors, Canice; and Gemperle, Rosemary. "Toward Dignity in Care: An In-service Model." *Death Education* 1 (Spring 1977): 113–30.

National Cancer Institute. Personal letter from Lawrence D. Burke, Program Director for Rehabilitation Treatment, Rehabilitation & Continuing Care Branch (DCCR), HEW, December 15, 1977.

National Hospice Organization. *Hospice in America*. New Haven: National Hospice Organization, n.d.

National Hospice Organization. "Hospice Standards." 4th draft. Distributed to members of the National Hospice Organization Standard and Accreditation Committee, August 1, 1978.

National Hospice Organization. "Preliminary Directory of the National Hospice Organization." New Haven: National Hospice Organization, 1978.

Nealon, Thomas F., Jr., ed. *Management of the Patient with Cancer*. Philadelphia: W. B. Saunders, 1965.

Netsky, Martin G. "Dying in a System of 'Good Care': Case Report and Analysis." *The Pharos of Alpha Omega Alpha* 39 (April 1976): 57–61.

Newsletter of the National Committee on the Treatment of Intractable Pain, Washington, D.C., no. 1 (January 1978).

New York State Senate. Personal letter from Hugh T. Farley, Senator. December 9, 1977.

Nightingale, Florence. *Notes on Hospitals.* 3rd ed. London: Longman, Green, 1863.

1978 Cancer Facts and Figures. New York: American Cancer Society, 1977.

"1979 Federal Health Budget Analysis." *The Nation's Health* (Supplement), March 1978, pp. 5–12.

Norbeck, Edward. *Religion in Primitive Society.* New York: Harper and Row, 1961.

Noyes, Russell, Jr. and Travis, Terry A. "The Care of Terminally Ill Patients." *Archives of Internal Medicine* 132 (October 1973): 607–11.

Opler, M. E. "Further Comparative Anthropological Data Bearing on the Solution of a Psychological Problem." *Journal of Social Psychology* 9 (1938): 477–84.

________. "An Interpretation of Ambivalence of Two American Indian Tribes." *Journal of Social Psychology* 7 (1936): 82–115.

Organization of the Government of Canada, 1976. Toronto: Canadian Minister of Supply and Services, 1976.

O'Rourke, Rev. K. D. "Active and Passive Euthanasia: The Ethical Distinctions." *Hospital Progress* 57 (November 1976): 68–73.

Palliative Care Service: October 1976 Report. Montreal: Royal Victoria Hospital, McGill University, 1976.

Pascoe, Jean. "He Manages the Final Rites." *Prism* 3 (June 1975): 62–4.

Patrick, Jane Gassner. "Should the Doctor Decide Whether You Live or Die?" *New West* 2 (December 19, 1977): 50–52 ff.

Pattison, E. Mansell, ed. *The Experience of Dying.* Englewood Cliffs, New Jersey: Prentice-Hall, 1977.

Pellman, Donald R. "Learning To Live with Dying." *New York Times Magazine,* December 5, 1976.

Perlberg, Mark. "The Dressing of the Graves." *Prism* 3 (June 1975): 50–53.

Phillips, D. F. "The Hospital and the Dying Patient." *Hospitals* 46 (February 1972): 68 et passim.

Plant, Janet. "Finding a Home for Hospice Care in the United States." *Hospitals* 51 (July 1, 1977): 53–62.

"A Primer on Brompton's Cocktail." Report prepared by Methodist Hospital of Indiana, Inc., Indianapolis, n.d.

Quinlan, Joseph and Julia, with Phyllis Battelle. *Karen Ann.* Garden City, New York: Doubleday, 1977.

Quintana, Jose B. "Health Care and the Moral Consensus: A Study of the Legal Implications of the Euthanasia of the Terminally Ill Patient." Master's thesis, Duke University, 1974.

Reinbach, Andrew. "'Brain Death': An Issue That Won't Die." *Health Care Week* 1 (February 13, 1978): 8.

Reynolds, D. K. and Kalish, Richard. "The Social Ecology of Dying: Observations of Wards for the Terminally Ill." *Hospital and Community Psychiatry* 25 (March 1974): 147–52.

The Right To Die with Dignity: A Discussion of the Medical, Legal and Ethical Aspects of Euthanasia. Remarks and discussion at the First Euthanasia Conference of the Euthanasia Educational Fund. New York: The Euthanasia Educational Council, November 23, 1968.

"Right-to-Die Law Runs into Problems." *Los Angeles Times,* November 25, 1977, part II, p. 9.

"Riverside Awarded NCI Contract." *Newsletter of the National Hospice Organization* 1 (November 1977).

Rose, M. A. and Pories, Walter J. "Some Additional Notes on Hospice." *Ohio State Medical Journal* 73 (June 1977): 379–82.

Rosenkranz, Samuel. *The Meaning in Your Life*. New York: Philosophical Library, 1958.

Rosner, F. "Prolonging Life or Prolonging Dying." *JAMA* 229 (July 1, 1974): 25.

Rosner, Fred. *Studies in Torah Judaism: Modern Medicine and Jewish Law*. New York: Yeshiva University, 1972.

Rossman, Parker. *Hospice: Creating New Models of Care for the Terminally Ill*. New York: Association Press, 1977.

Rozovsky, Lorne E. "Death, Dead Bodies and the Law." *Canadian Hospital,* July 1970, pp. 52–5.

Rozovsky, Lorne E. "The Moment of Death." *Canadian Hospital,* September 1972, pp. 24–5.

_________. "Resuscitation and the Euthanasia Debate." *Dimensions in Health Service* 52 (November 1975): 8–9.

Rubin, Enid. "Marin Hospice: Answering the Prayers of the Terminally Ill." *Mill Valley Record,* May 4, 1977.

Rubin, Philip, ed. *Clinical Oncology for Medical Students and Physicians*. 4th ed. Rochester, N.Y.: American Cancer Society, 1974.

Russell, O. Ruth. *Freedom To Die*. New York: Human Sciences Press, 1975.

St. Christopher's Hospice. "Annual Report, 1973–74." London: St. Christopher's Hospice, 1974.

St. Christopher's Hospice. "Annual Report, 1976–77." London: St. Christopher's Hospice, 1977.

St. Christopher's Hospice. "Details of Admissions and Discharges During 1975." Mimeographed. London: St. Christopher's Hospice, 1976.

Sampson, Wallace J. "Dying at Home." *JAMA* 238 (November 28, 1977): 2,405–06.

The Sanctity of Social Life: Physician's Treatment of Critically Ill Patients. New York: Russell Sage Foundation, 1975.

Satchell, Michael. "How To Enjoy Life—Up to the Last Moment." *Parade,* October 16, 1977.

Saunders, Cicely. "Care for the Dying." *Patient Care* 3 (June 1976).

_________. "The Challenge of Terminal Care." *Scientific Foundations of Oncology*. Edited by T. Symington and R. L. Carter. London: William Heinemann Medical Books, Ltd., n.d.

_________. "The Last Stages of Life." *American Journal of Nursing* 65 (March 1965): 70–5.

_________. "The Need for In-Patient Care for the Patient with Terminal Cancer." *Middlesex Hospital Journal* 72 (February 1973).

———. "St. Christopher's Hospice." London: St. Christopher's Hospice, 1977.

Scherzer, C. J. *Ministering to the Dying*. Englewood Cliffs, New Jersey: Prentice-Hall, 1963.

Schnaper, L. A. et al. "Euthanasia: An Overview." *Maryland State Medical Journal* 26 (March 1977): 42–8.

Schoenberg, Bernard et al., eds. *Anticipatory Grief*. New York: Columbia University Press, 1974.

Schulz, R. "Meeting the Three Major Needs of the Dying Patient." *Geriatrics* 31 (June 1976): 107–10.

Scott, Patricia Cumin. *Some Information for Those Caring for Patients*. London: St. Christopher's Hospice, 1974.

Seldon, Elaine. ". . . Even the Elderly." *RN*, January, 1976.

Selkurt, Ewald E. "Death." *World Book Encyclopedia*, 1967.

Selltiz, Claire; Wrightsman, Lawrence; and Cook, Stuart. *Research Methods in Social Relations*. 3rd ed. New York: Holt, Rinehart and Winston, 1976.

Shaffer, Helen B. "Right to Death." *Editorial Research Reports* 1 (January 27, 1978): 62–80.

Sharpe, Gilbert. "Euthanasia: The Consequences of Turning Off the Respirator." *Canadian Lawyer*, December 1977, pp. 8–9.

Shephard, D. A. "Terminal Care: Towards An Ideal." *Canadian Medical Association Journal* 115 (July 17, 1976): 97–8 ff.

Shimken, Michael B. *Science and Cancer*. HEW Publication No. (NIH) 74-568, 2nd rev. National Cancer Institute. Washington, D.C.: U.S. Government Printing Office, 1973.

Shneidman, Edwin S., ed. *Death: Current Perspectives*. Palo Alto, California: Mayfield, 1976.

Shneidman, Edwin S. *Deaths of Man*. Baltimore: Penguin, 1974.

Slater, E. "Assisted Suicide—Some Ethical Considerations," *International Journal of Health Service* 6 (November 2, 1976): 321–30.

Snider, Arthur J. "LSD for the Terminally Ill?" *Los Angeles Times*, May 12, 1978, part IV, pp. 8–9.

Snider, Arthur J. and Gould, Donald W. "Health and Disease, General Overview." *1977 Yearbook, Covering the Year 1976*. Chicago: Encyclopaedia Britanicca, 1977.

Somerville, R. M. "Death Education As Part of Family Life Education: Using Imaginative Literature for Insights into Family Crisis." *The Family Coordinator* 20 (1971): 209–24.

"Standards For Cardiopulmonary Resuscitation and Emergency Cardiac Care." *JAMA* (Supplement) 227 (February 18, 1974): 833–68.

Stevens, Roland. "Euthanasia: A Doctor Speaks . . ." Address delivered at organizing meeting of the Euthanasia Educational Fund, Rochester, New York chapter, February 4, 1971.

Stinchcomb, Ethel M. "A Study of the Attitudes of Graduate Nurses Toward the Direct Care of the Terminally ill Patient." Ed. D. dissertation, University of Maryland, 1969.

Stoddard, Sandol. *The Hospice Movement: A Better Way of Caring for the Dying*. Briarcliff Manor, New York: Stein & Day, 1978.

Strugnell, C. *Adjustment to Widowhood and Some Related Problems: A Selective and Annotated Bibliography*. New York: Health Sciences, 1973.

Sudnow, David. *Passing On: The Social Organization of Dying*. Englewood Cliffs, New Jersey: Prentice-Hall, 1967.

Summers, Dorothy H. and Young, Joan M. *To Comfort Always*. London: St. Christopher's Hospice, n.d.

Sumner, William G. and Keller, Albert. *The Science of Society*. New Haven: Yale University Press, 1927.

Supreme Court of New Jersey. Decision in the Matter of Karen Quinlan, an alleged incompetent, argued January 26, 1976, decided March 31, 1976.

Tagge, Garth. "Critical Care: A Classification System for ICU Patients." *The Hospital Medical Staff* 5 (February 1976): 1–6.

Taylor, Carol. "Death, American Style." *Death Education* 1 (Summer 1977): 177–85.

Terminal Care For Cancer Patients. Chicago: The Central Service for the Chronically Ill of the Institute of Medicine of Chicago, 1950.

"Terminal Care: Connecticut Corporation Will Build a Hospital for the Dying." *Modern Healthcare* 2 (July 1974): 101.

"Terminal Patients and 'No Code' Orders." *Regan Report on Nursing Law* 14 (November 1973): 1.

Traska, Maria. "Hillhaven Negotiates For NCI Grant." *Modern Healthcare* 7 (September 1977): 40–1.

"Treating Patients in Their Homes—Often Cheaper, Often Better." *U.S. News & World Report*, October 25, 1976, p. 73.

Triche, Charles W., III, and Triche, D. S. *The Euthanasia Controversy, 1812–1974: A Bibliography with Selected Annotations*. Troy, New York: Whitston, 1975.

Trubo, Richard. *An Act of Mercy: Euthanasia Today*. Los Angeles: NASH, 1973.

Twycross, Robert G. "Address to the National Committee on the Treatment of Intractable Pain, Jan. 31, 1978, Washington, D.C." *Newsletter of the National Committee on the Treatment of Intractable Pain* 1 (March 1978): 1–2.

__________. "Studies on the Use of Diamorphine in Advanced Malignant Disease." M.D. dissertation, University of Oxford, 1976.

__________. "The Use of Diamorphine in the Management of Terminal Cancer." *Journal of Thanatology* 2 (Summer-Fall 1972): 733–43.

__________. "The Use of Narcotic Analgesics in Terminal Illness." *Journal of Medical Ethics* 1 (1975): 11–17.

U.S., Congress, House, Committee on Interstate and Foreign Commerce, Subcommittee on Health and the Environment. *A Discursive Dictionary of Health Care*. 94th Congress, 2nd Session, February 1976.

U.S., Department of Commerce, Bureau of Economic Analysis. *The National Income and Product Accounts of the U.S., 1929–74, Statistical Tables*. Washington, D.C.: Government Printing Office, 1977.

U.S., Department of HEW. "Medicare and Medicaid Hospice Projects." *Federal Register* 43, no. 209 (October 27, 1978): 50,376–8.

U.S., Department of HEW, Public Health Service, National Center for Health Statistics. *Episodes and Duration of Hospitalization in the Last Year of Life, U.S., 1961*, Series 22, no. 2. Washington, D.C.: Government Printing Office, 1966.

U.S., Department of HEW, Public Health Service, National Center for Health Statistics. *Hospitalization in the Last Year of Life-1961*, Series 22, no. 1. Washington, D.C.: Government Printing Office, 1965.

U.S., Department of HEW, Public Health Service, Health Resources Administration, National Center for Health Statistics. *Vital Statistics of the United States, 1971*, Vol. II—Mortality, part A. Rockville, Maryland: Government Printing Office, 1975.

U.S., Public Health Service. *Vital Statistics of the United States, 1958*, Vol. II. Washington, D.C.: Government Printing Office, 1960.

Vaisrub, Samuel. "Afterthoughts on Afterlife." *Archives of Internal Medicine* 137 (February 1977): 150.

van Till, H. A. H. "Diagnosis of Death in Comatose Patients under Resuscitation Treatment: A Critical Review of the Harvard Report." *American Journal of Law and Medicine* 2 (Summer 1976): 1–40.

Veith, Frank et al. "Brain Death: I. A Status Report of Medical & Ethical Considerations." *JAMA* 238 (October 10, 1977): 1,651–5.

__________. "Brain Death: II. A Status Report of Legal Considerations." *JAMA* 238 (October 17, 1977): 1,744–8.

Vellucci, Matthew J. et al., comps. *The National Directory of State Agencies, 1974–1975*. Washington, D.C.: Information Resources Press, 1974.

Vere, Duncan W. *Voluntary Euthanasia—Is There an Alternative?* London: Christian Medical Fellowship, 1971.

Vernick, J. J. *Selected Bibliography on Death and Dying*. Bethesda, Maryland: National Institute of Child Health and Human Development, 1971.

Vernon, Glenn M. *Sociology of Death*. New York: Ronald Press, 1970.

Vincent, R. H. "California Natural Death Act—Some Help with Antidysthanasia." *Journal of the Medical Association of Georgia* 66 (January 1977): 38–40.

von Hoffman, Nicholas. "Where Can We Die in Peace?" *Los Angeles Times*, May 29, 1978.

Waldman, A. M. "Medical Ethics and the Hopelessly Ill Child." *Journal of Pediatrics* 88 (May 1976): 890–2.

Wallis, Wilson D. "Transmigration of the Soul." *World Book Encyclopedia*, 1967.

Walshe, W. G. "Death and Disposal of the Dead: Chinese." *Hasting's Encyclopedia of Religion and Ethics*. New York: Charles Scribner's, 1911.

Walter, Norman T. "The Coming of Death in America: Concepts in Transition." Mimeographed, July 15, 1976.

Walters, Susan, ed. *Canadian Almanac and Directory, 1977*. Toronto: Copp Clark, 1977.

Ward, A. W. M. "Terminal Care Homes." *Hospital and Health Services Review* 71 (July 1975): 233–6.

Wass, Hannelore, ed. *Death Education* 2, nos. 1–2 (Spring/Summer 1978). Special Issue on The Hospice.

"Ways of Looking at Death: Bio-Ethics and Public Policy II." Conference sponsored by the National Conference of Christians and Jews at University of California-Los Angeles, January 17, 1978.

"We Who Stand At the Border of Life and Death." Interview with Robert Jay Lifton. *Prism* 3 (June 1975): 46–49 ff.

Weaver, Peter. "Hospices Ease Pain of Dying." *Los Angeles Times*, part VIII, May 7, 1978, p. 16.

Wehrwein, Austin. "Should 'Brain Death' Definitions Be Law? Yes." *Health Care Week* 1 (February 13, 1978): 9.

Wentzel, K. B. "The Dying Are the Living." *American Journal of Nursing* 76 (June 1976): 956–7.

West, T. S. "Approach to Death." *Nursing Mirror*, Oct. 10, 1974.

__________. "Hospice Care for a Dying Person and His Family." Paper presented at the First International Conference on Patient Counselling, Amsterdam, April 1976.

Whitman, H. H. and Lukes, S. J. "Behavior Modification for Terminally Ill Patients." *American Journal of Nursing* 75 (January 1975): 155–7.

Wilkes, E. "Terminal Care and the Special Nursing Unit." *Nursing Times* 71 (January 9, 1975): 57–9.

Will, George F. "A Good Death." *Newsweek*, January 9, 1978, p. 72.

Wolper, Lawrence F. *Death and Euthanasia: Man's Continuing Dilemma*. New York: Bernard M. Baruch College, City University of New York, 1973.

"Woman Dies After Life Support Equipment Is Disconnected." *Valley News* (San Fernando Valley, Calif.), December 28, 1977.

Woodson, Robert. "The Concept of Hospice Care in Terminal Disease." *Breast Cancer*. Edited by J. M. Vaeth, Basel, Switzerland: Karger, 1976, pp. 161–79.

Woodward, Kenneth L. et al. "Living with Dying." *Newsweek*, May 1, 1978, pp. 52–61.

Worcester, A. *The Care of the Aged, the Dying, and the Dead*. Springfield: Thomas, 1935.

Xiques, Linda. "Dying at Home." *Pacific Sun*, January 28–February 3, 1977.

Yalom, Irvin D. and Greaves, Carlos. "Group Therapy with the Terminally Ill." *American Journal of Psychiatry* 134 (April 1977): 396–400.

Zorza, Victor and Zorza, Rosemary. "The Death of a Daughter." *Washington Post*, Outlook section, January 22, 1978.

Index

B

C

D

E

F

G

H

M

N

O

P

About the Author

Kenneth P. Cohen is presently the administrator of Van Nuys Community Hospital, Van Nuys, California. He received his Ph.D. in business administration (health services management) from California Western University, Santa Ana, California and his Master of Public Health degree from the University of California, Los Angeles. A hospital chief executive officer for the past 14 years, he has been active in a number of hospital organizations, serving on various boards. Currently, Dr. Cohen is chairman of the legislative committee of the Southern California Regional Hospice Association, and he serves as vice chairman of the malpractice and insurance committee of the National Hospice Organization.